Everything You Always Wanted to Know About

PUBERTY

—and Shouldn't Be Googling

FOR CURIOUS BOYS

BY MORRIS KATZ *(who just barely made it out the other side)*

ILLUSTRATED BY AMELIA PINNEY

downtown bookworks

downtown bookworks

Downtown Bookworks Inc.
New York, New York
www.downtownbookworks.com

Special thanks to Dez Lasseter, Juliette Palermo,
and Kevin Duval for their helpful feedback.

Thank you to Amelia and Georgia for
making this book so beautiful,
to Hannah for tolerating me,
to my brothers for all of the material,
to my dad for the R-rated jokes
I had to cut—and of course,
to my mom, for everything.
—MORRIS

Thanks to my grandmother, Shirley Kane,
who nurtures creativity.
—AMELIA

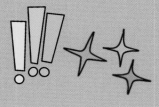

what's in this book

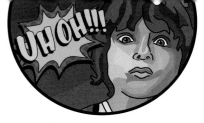

PART 1

PART 2

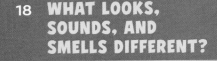

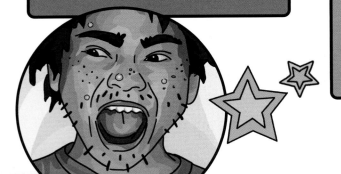

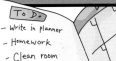

PART 3

YEAH!

POPCORN POPCO

foreword

This isn't the puberty textbook your parents read in Stone Age health class. This isn't the embarrassing body book your single, out-of-town aunt sends you on the wrong birthday. And it isn't written by some 50-year-old doctor who maybe didn't realize how creepy it was to write a book explaining puberty to a bunch of little boys. This is something much, much better (and a lot less weird). I'm going to tell you about all of the crazy, exciting changes your body and brain are going through—and it's going to be fun!

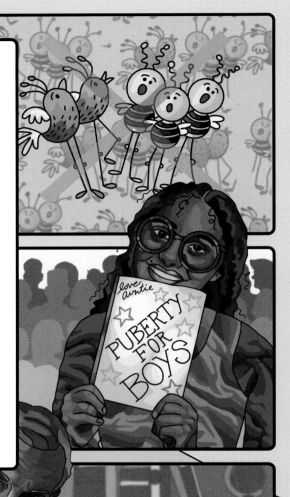

Who am I to tell you this stuff? My name is Morris. I'm 21 years old, and I have three younger brothers, so I'm used to explaining things. I've just barely escaped the grasp of puberty. I still get pimples! And I hardly have any chest hair—yet. When I was in middle school, I learned about puberty from the internet and from my friends (who knew exactly as little as I did). Everything I know now, I know because I lived through it. All of it! The months where I'd sleep, eat, and grow three inches. Countless surprise erections. Hairs sprouting in places where I'd become certain they would never emerge . . . or it never occurred to me that hair could grow. I had fits of hormonal rage and breakouts so bad I wondered if I was recognizable under all the acne.

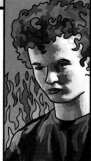

And I lived to tell the tale. As a recent puberty graduate, I wanted to write a book for my little brothers, and for all of you who have yet to serve your time and grow and transform in ways that are both harrowing and remarkable. I wanted to write the book I wish I could have turned to, instead of relying on my friend Noah. I hope you enjoy it—and learn something too.

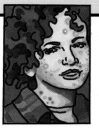
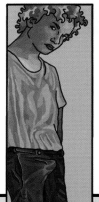
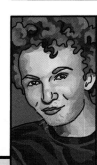
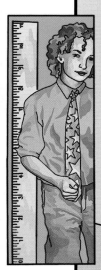

ASK FOR HELP...

This is a general overview of puberty, but as we'll talk about, everyone has his own unique experience of puberty. If I could write a book specifically tailored to each and every individual's experience, I would. However, I'm a little too busy to go around measuring growth spurts, counting hairs, and delving into each of your personal lives. I'll leave that important work to you, your pediatricians, and your therapists.

Because this isn't personalized for every reader, there may be gaps in the information you need. If you have questions, talk to a responsible adult in your life—your doctor, a parent or guardian, your older brother (who's hopefully as cool as I am). You're going to learn a lot from this book, but you won't learn everything. In certain places, this may be more of a conversation starter for deeper questions and conversations you want to have with people you trust.

ENOUGH ABOUT ME

As you read, you'll notice that my personal anecdotes reflect my own life: I was raised by a mom and dad in New York City, and I like girls. Those facts shaped my own experience, but that doesn't mean it's a universal experience, and it definitely doesn't mean that my heterosexual, cis male, traditional family, urban childhood is the standard, or better than anyone else's experience. (In fact, if you met my eighth grade girlfriend, you'd probably say it's worse.) The facts and information in the book should be useful to everyone, regardless of who you like, how you identify, or the color of your skin. My personal stories and views are shaped by who I am, just as I'm sure yours are too.

I refer to "boys" and "girls" throughout the book because that's generally how I speak, though I recognize that gender identity takes on many names and forms and pronouns and I mean no offense and hope to be inclusive. It is just the style we decided on so the book can feel conversational. Lastly, I refer to all of my brothers simply as "my brother" to protect their identities a tiny bit.

THE ATTACK OF THE HORMONES

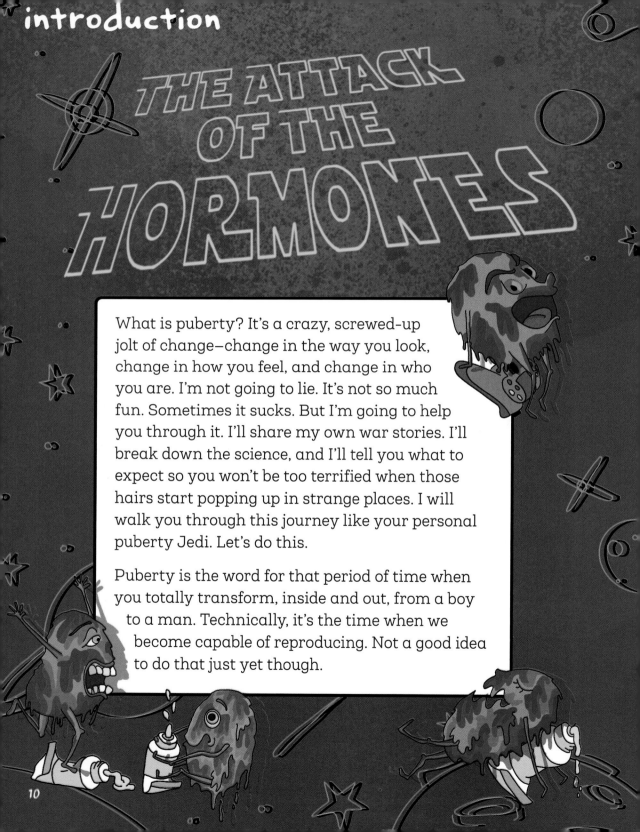

What is puberty? It's a crazy, screwed-up jolt of change—change in the way you look, change in how you feel, and change in who you are. I'm not going to lie. It's not so much fun. Sometimes it sucks. But I'm going to help you through it. I'll share my own war stories. I'll break down the science, and I'll tell you what to expect so you won't be too terrified when those hairs start popping up in strange places. I will walk you through this journey like your personal puberty Jedi. Let's do this.

Puberty is the word for that period of time when you totally transform, inside and out, from a boy to a man. Technically, it's the time when we become capable of reproducing. Not a good idea to do that just yet though.

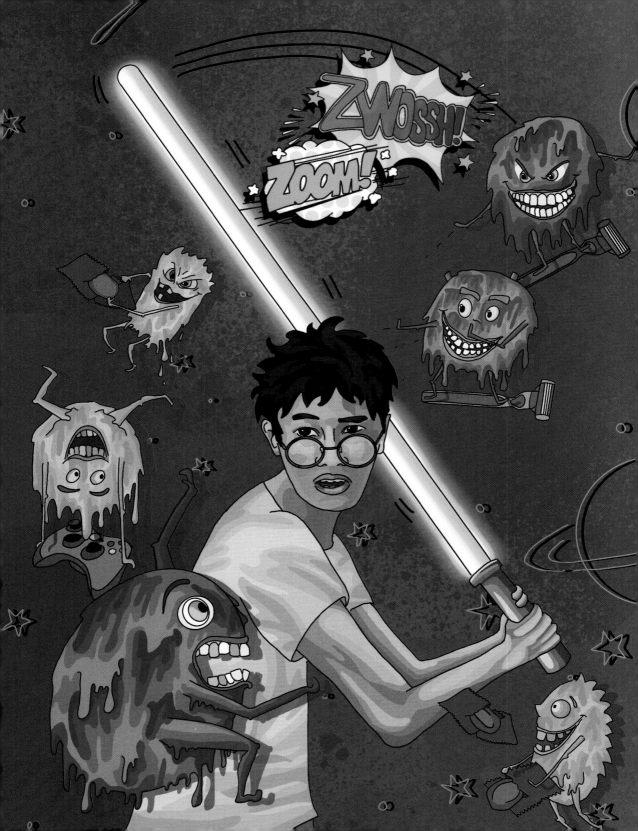

Puberty strikes different people at different times. For most boys, it kicks in sometime between the ages of 12 and 14 (though kids can start as early as 9). The summer after I turned 12, I slept 16 hours a night, ate 5 meals a day, and shot up 6 inches. One of my brothers didn't really start to transform until he was 14. He stressed out and worried about it every day of middle school, but he's 15 now and looking and sounding more and more like a man every day. Don't get too focused on *when* you will go through puberty, because, we all go through it sooner or later.

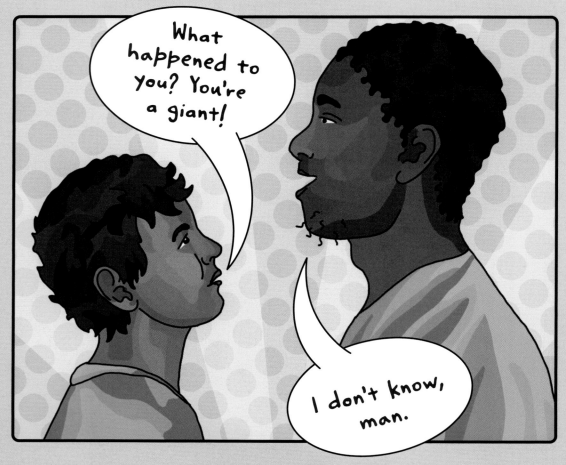

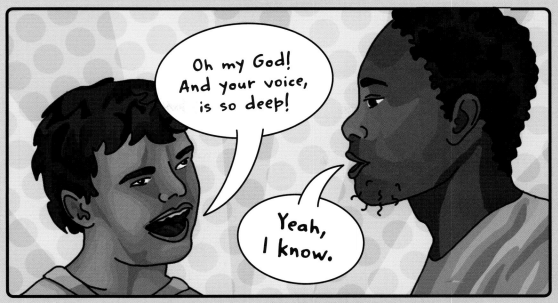

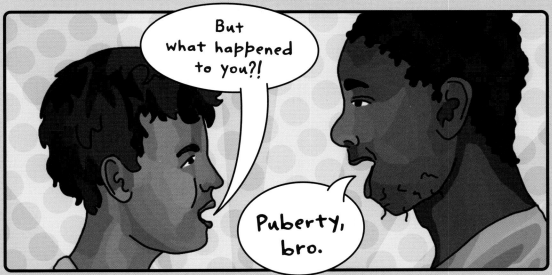

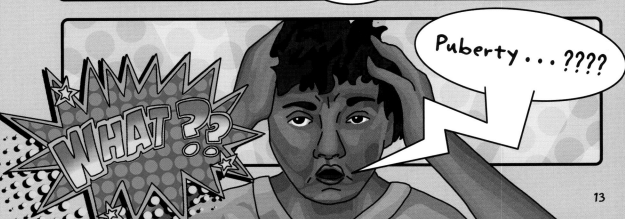

So what exactly triggers these insane changes? It's your *hormones* going crazy.

Hormones are like chemical messengers in our bodies. Let me see if I can explain this in a way that doesn't sound like a health class. If puberty is a car, hormones are the engine.

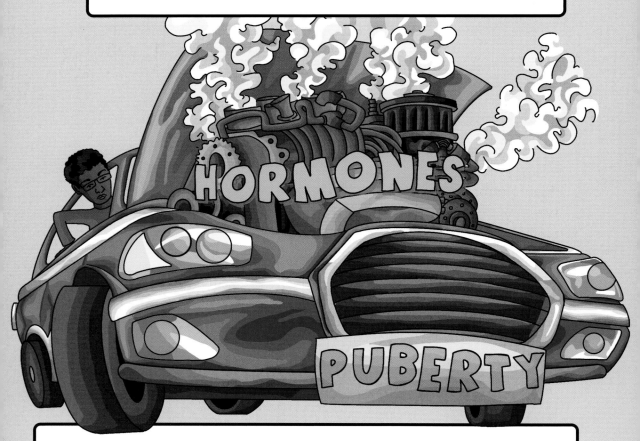

Puberty starts when your brain releases specific hormones that trigger your body's development. Basically, you get to a certain age, and your brain realizes that it's time for you to become a man, and it releases a puberty hormone called gonadotropin-releasing hormone. I don't know why scientists choose such complicated names for everything—thankfully, it's called GnRH for short.

GnRH rushes through the body so it can get to the pituitary gland (a pea-sized gland that's located at the base of the brain). This gland gets the message that "it's puberty time" from our buddy GnRH. (Woo! Woo!) Then it releases two *more* puberty hormones: luteinizing hormone (LH, for short) and follicle-stimulating hormone (FSH).

LH and FSH disperse throughout the body and trigger the production of testosterone in your testicles. They start this as early as age 9, but you won't even realize anything is different for a few years while the hormones are working behind the scenes. Testosterone is the hormone that causes most of the changes a boy goes through during puberty. When you're a teenager, you'll have more testosterone in your body than at any other point in your life. In addition to generating testosterone, the release of FSH and LH starts your body's production of sperm. Sperm cells enable men to reproduce (though hopefully, you won't be worrying about that for a while).

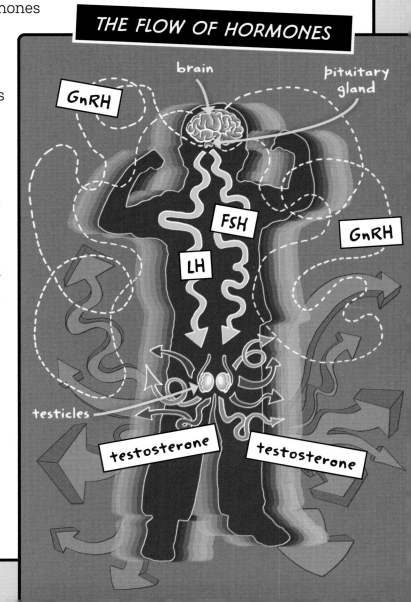

THE FLOW OF HORMONES

brain

pituitary gland

GnRH

FSH

LH

GnRH

testicles

testosterone

testosterone

During the earliest stage of puberty, your hormones are just getting to work, and you won't really be able to see any changes. When the physical changes start to happen, they will *roughly* follow this timeline. It's important to remember that this is just a guideline—hormones affect everybody in different ways and at different times. You could get a really deep voice but not a lot of facial hair. Your penis could grow years before the rest of your body does, or vice versa. Don't worry. If you are a boy now, you will become a man soon enough.

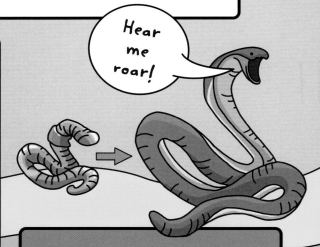

Hear me roar!

AROUND AGE 11
(maybe sooner, maybe later):

- **The testicles and scrotum (skin around the testicles) start to grow.**

- **You may start to see a tiny bit of pubic hair at the base of the penis.**

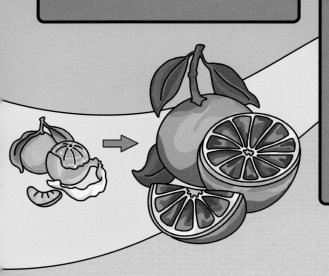

AROUND AGE 13:

- **Your penis gets longer.**

- **Your voice begins to crack.**

- **Wet dreams start.**

- **Your muscles get larger.**

- **Your growth spurt begins.**

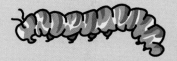

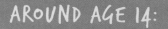

AROUND AGE 14:

- **Your penis, testicles, and scrotum continue to get bigger, and the scrotum gets darker.**

- **Armpit hair starts to grow.**

- **Acne appears.**

- **Your voice deepens for good.**

- **Facial hair starts to sprout.**

Over the next few years, you look, sound, and smell more and more like a man

✱At first, we were going to use images of my penis to get this point across but the publisher said it was inappropriate so here we are, with some fruit and animal metaphors. Is your penis actually going to become an animal or fruit? No. Probably not. What will happen during puberty is your penis will develop and transform. You guys are smart though, you get the point.

Now that we have a sense of what gets puberty going (and why), let's take a look at the changes brought on by this sudden flood of hormones in your body.

PART 1

WHAT LOOKS, SOUNDS, AND SMELLS DIFFERENT?

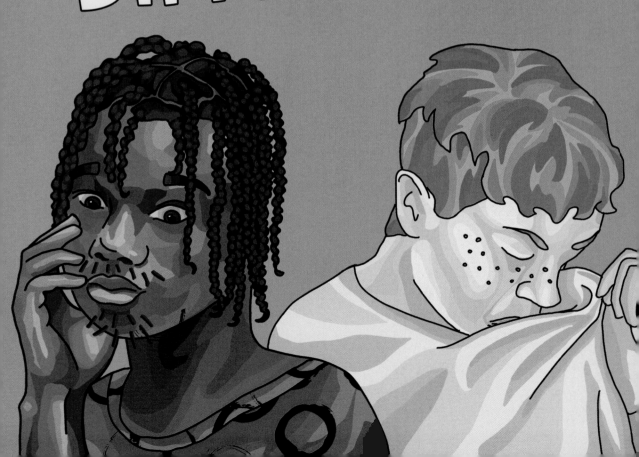

By the time you've gone through puberty, you'll be way taller than you were before. Your voice will be deeper. You'll sweat more, and you'll be hairier. Most exciting of all, your penis will be bigger than it was before. These changes are great and they're a natural, normal part of your development. But, there are a lot of them happening at once, so we're going to try to break it down one change at a time. We'll start off with what's going to look different.

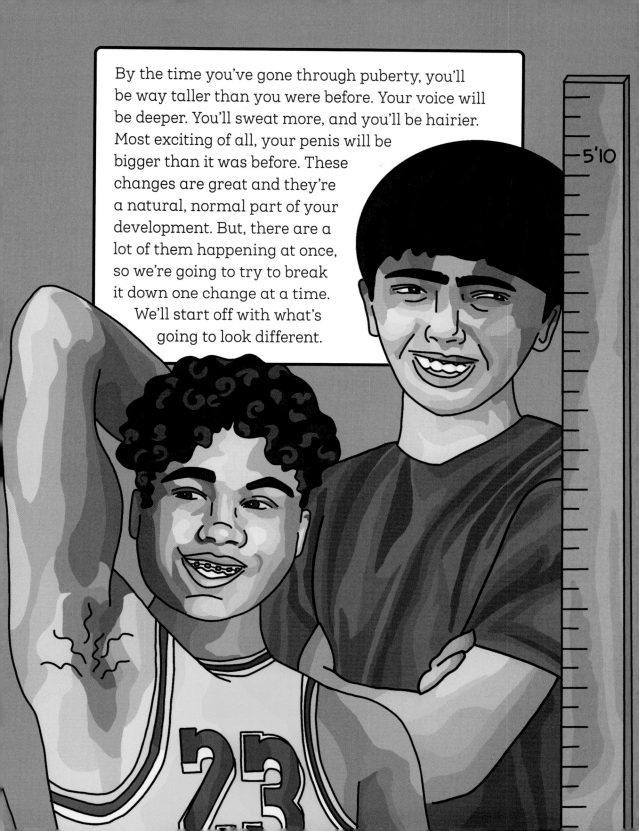

"You Got So TALL!"

Pre-puberty, you're kid-size. You're like a McDonalds Happy Meal. You come in a cute little box with a toy. Post-puberty, you're a Big Mac, baby! You might even pass your parents in height (that part is really fun)! From the time you're about four until you hit puberty, you grow about 2 inches per year. When puberty strikes, you will grow about 3 to 5 inches each year.

Nice.

BOOM

!?

POW

Along the way to your new height there can be growing pains (both figuratively and literally).

One of my brothers had physical growing pains. He felt achey all over because of the rate at which his boy body was being stretched into a man's body. You may also go through a clumsy period. Your arms, legs, hands, and feet grow faster than your torso. So, in addition to making you look odd, the growth can be so rapid that it takes a while for your coordination to catch up to your new center of gravity.

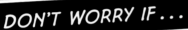

DON'T WORRY IF...

. . . girls seem to be towering over you. Girls typically get their growth spurts before boys do. For a brief period of time, girls may have a bit of a height advantage. But then boys grow more during puberty, and that's when they often become taller than girls their age. Though not always. Either way, don't sweat it— there's nothing wrong with being shorter than a girl!

. . . your body is aching. You're not breaking, you're just growing.

. . . you appear to thicken before you stretch out. When puberty kicks off, your body starts to store extra fat. This is totally normal.

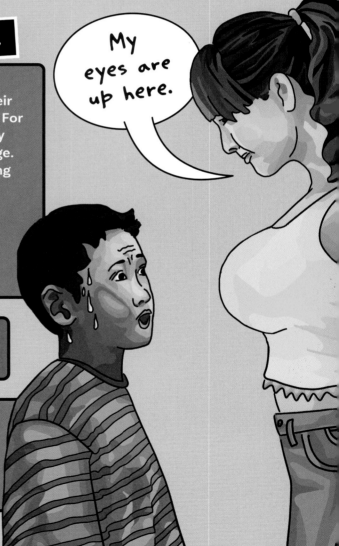

My eyes are up here.

How's the View from UP THERE?

What's different now that you're tall? Well, other than the fact that you'll constantly have to hear about "how much you've grown" at family gatherings and your jeans and sweatpants won't cover your ankles anymore, you'll notice an adjustment period. It's like you've been switched into a different body—a new body that you don't have as solid a grasp on yet. At times, you might feel clumsy and uncomfortable, but in due time, you'll start to excel with your new and improved body. As Uncle Ben said to Peter Parker, "With great power comes great responsibility." (I'm a bit of a geek so we may come back to this quote more than once before this book is over.) Be conscious that you're bigger than you used to be, man-sized even. As my mother pointed out to me one time soon after my growth spurt, when I was wrestling with one of my brothers, "You're like an adult beating up a child now." For a while, on the inside you'll still feel like a boy. The thing is, in your new body, the world will see you as a man.

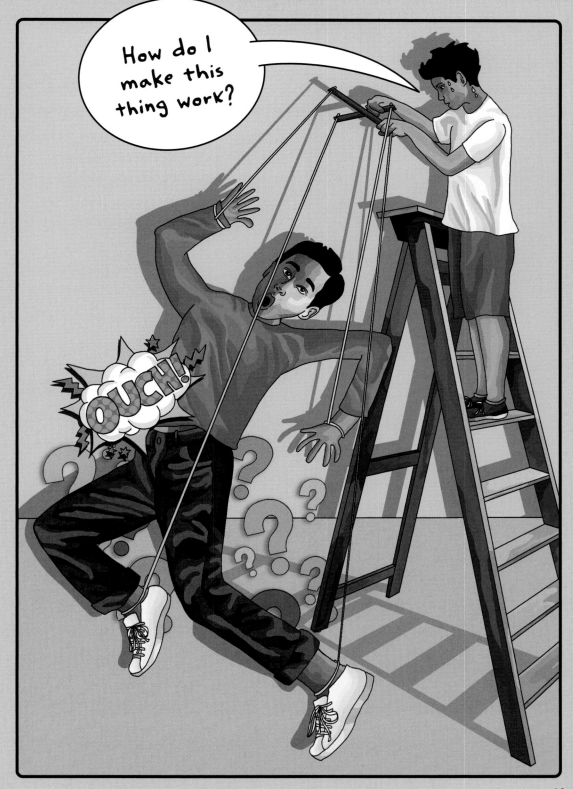

Big Boy STRENGTH

Not only do you get taller, but you also get stronger.

Notice your body starting to get a little toned? Getting some real muscles? What's happening? Have you been bitten by a radioactive spider or exposed to gamma rays like Spider-Man and the Incredible Hulk?

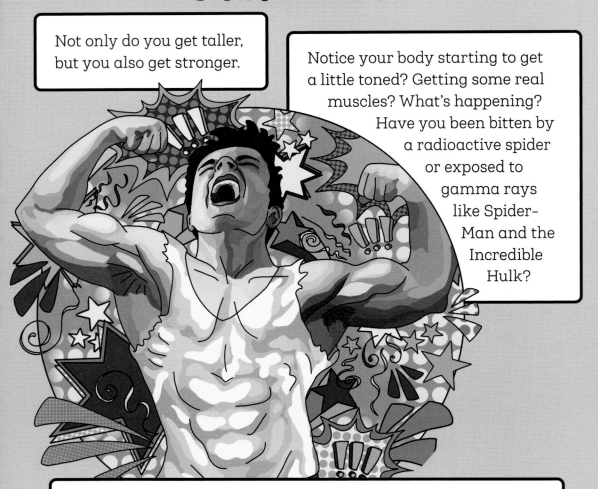

Unfortunately it's neither. You're not going through a superhero transition, it's just good ol' puberty striking again. Testosterone helps increase muscle mass. If you've dreamed of having big biceps, now's your chance. If you play competitive sports, you will really start to feel the benefits of your new muscles.

Everyone loses fat deposits at a different rate, and muscle growth varies from boy to boy as well. Nobody gets superhero-ripped overnight. But your shape will definitely start to change.

FUELING UP

Because you're getting bigger and stronger, you will also be way hungrier. As a teenager, I usually ate five meals a day, and so did my brothers. Cut us a break—it's not easy growing taller and growing hair and growing body parts! The summer of my growth spurt, practically all I did when I wasn't eating was drink milk and sleep.

When you're that hungry, it's easy to shove anything edible down your throat. But it's a good time to start paying attention to what's going into your body. You will actually feel much better if you eat well. That means filling up on protein (meat, eggs, beans, nuts), fruit, and vegetables—not chips and cookies. Good nutrition improves your skin, your mood, and your physical health. Think of yourself as a hibernating bear. You'll eat more than you've ever eaten before, and you'll sleep more than you've ever slept. Sleep, eat, grow. Sleep, eat, grow. Repeat.

Pre-puberty, I used to wake up at 6 a.m. and run into the living room to watch *SportsCenter* before anyone else in the house woke up. Once puberty hit, it took a team of Navy SEALs to get me out of bed before 10. It's important to listen to your body. Give it the rest and the sustenance it wants.

HUNGRY, HUNGRY ~~HIPPOS~~ BOYS

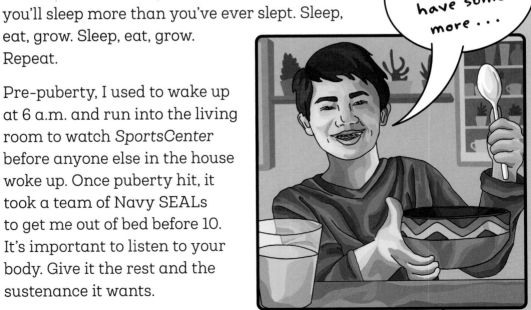

Please sir, may I have some more . . .

Your NEW Penis

This is the big one (no pun intended). One of the main changes triggered by puberty is penis growth. Over the course of a few years, your penis will get longer and bigger. Puberty is, in large part, the chemical process in which you become a "man" in the scientific sense of the word. In other words, you become capable of reproducing. And the penis is the vehicle for reproduction.

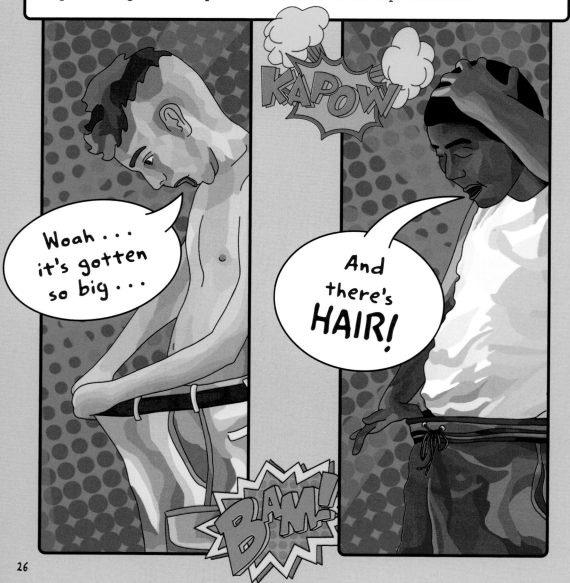

TESTICLES AND SCROTUM

During puberty, your testicles (balls) start to produce sperm all the time. They are like a 24-hour sperm factory—one that will stay open for the rest of your life. Your testicles are also busy producing testosterone. In many people, one testicle is higher than the other. Sometimes they hang evenly.

The scrotum, the sac around the testicles, gets very busy during puberty, too. Its muscles move the sperm in your testicles around to keep it at the right temperature. The surge of testosterone can cause your scrotum to get darker during puberty. Some people also get tiny bumps on the skin of the scrotum. All of these changes are completely normal, and nothing to worry about.

UPS AND DOWNS

When your body is warm, your scrotum hangs longer, and when you're cold, it pulls closer to the body. This happens to regulate the temperature of your sperm.

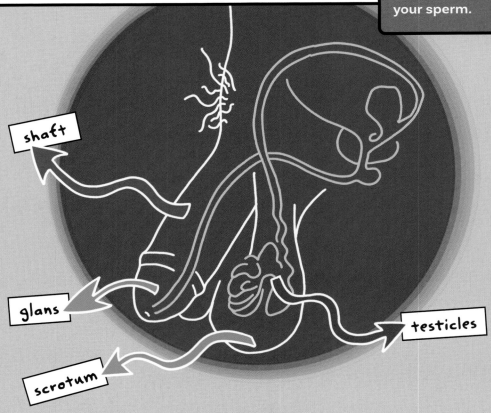

shaft

glans

testicles

scrotum

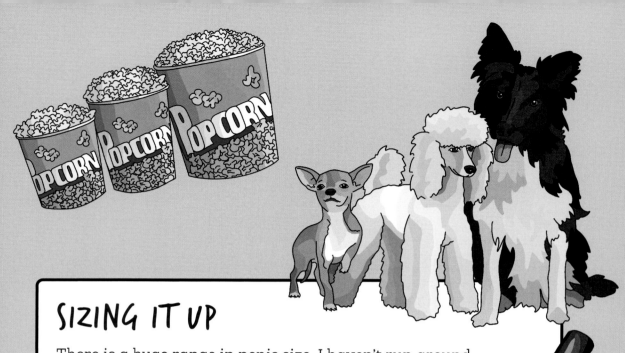

SIZING IT UP

There is a huge range in penis size. I haven't run around measuring, but I read that the average penis can be anywhere from 2.5 to 5 inches long when soft and 5 to 7 inches long when hard or erect. There's a myth that having a big penis is somehow significant and a test of your manliness. This is not true. For some people there is a big difference in size when the penis goes from soft to hard. For others, there's not a significant difference. Any which way, it's all totally normal. And regardless of the size of your penis, it'll serve its purpose when the time comes.

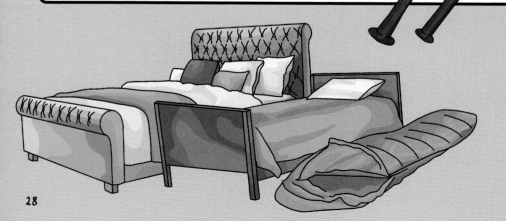

Before your penis begins to grow, something else will begin to grow...

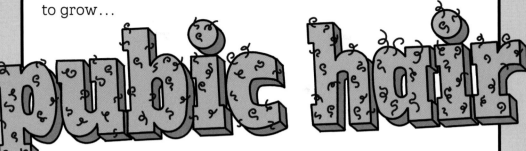

Pubic hair serves a purpose (other than freaking you out when it first starts sprouting). The genital area is rather sensitive, and pubic hair helps protect the goods. It prevents friction and keeps bacteria out. Pubic hair can feel awkward. ("Why the hell is there hair on my penis?") But it really isn't anything to be ashamed of. And eventually, as with all the other aspects of your new body, you'll get used to it.

TIME FOR A TRIM?

You probably go to a barber to get your haircut. But down there, you're on your own. Some people like to trim their pubic hair all the time, maybe even keeping it shaved, while others let it grow, only occasionally trimming it. As with the hair on your head, it's really about what you want and what makes you comfortable. My only real advice on the matter? Be careful down there! Your penis (all penises) are highly sensitive, and the last thing you want to do is cut yourself while going for a pubic hair mohawk (not something people actually do).

Armpit HAIR

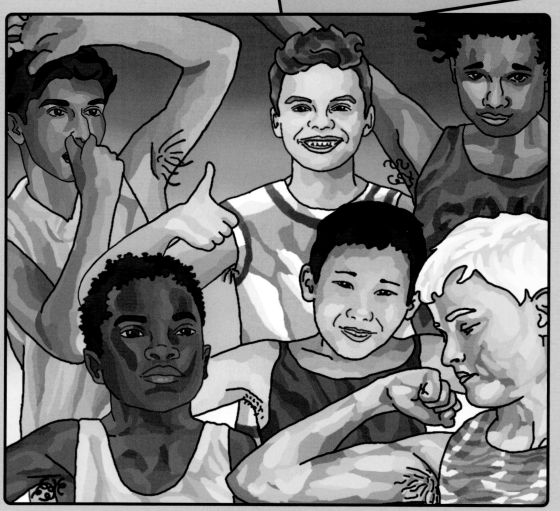

Armpit hair is a different experience for everyone. I liked my armpits as they were, smooth and hairless. My brother, on the other hand, checked his pits every day, eagerly awaiting the arrival of that first hair.

Armpit hair doesn't actually sprout in most boys until pretty far along in puberty. Before you hit the armpit hair milestone, your penis will have grown larger, and you'll probably have pubic hair and some muscles. You will be used to all kinds of changes, and then the armpit hair arrives. It doesn't always go in this order, but typically armpit hair comes in the later stages of puberty.

Some boys get just a few wiry strands, and others might have a thick bush. The one thing we all have in common though, is that it can get pretty smelly in there. Hair can stay wet when you sweat so more bacteria can live there, and that leads to more odor.

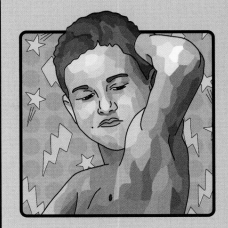

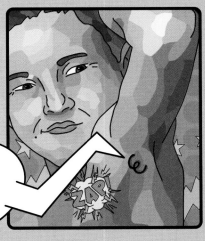

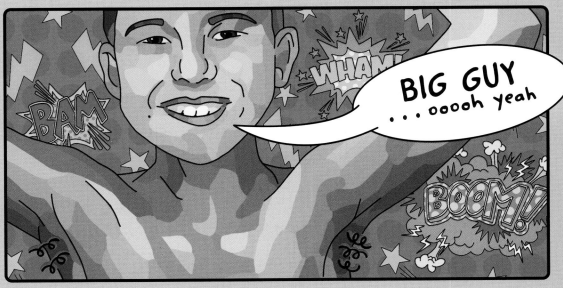

SWEATY Dayz

Boy, do I miss the days when I could run out of the house without worrying about whether or not I'd already put on deodorant. You think you sweat now? Just wait until puberty grabs a hold of you. You'll start sweating more and, worst of all, your sweat won't be the sweet, innocent, scentless liquid droplets you're used to, it'll be smelly as hell. That awful smell you might have noticed when your hairy uncle played basketball with you, or every time you walked into the locker room? That's your bedroom now. That's the scent that follows you around like a cloud and encourages friends to socially distance whether or not there's a pandemic.

So, what do you do? Well, I'm pleased to introduce you to my good friend, deodorant.

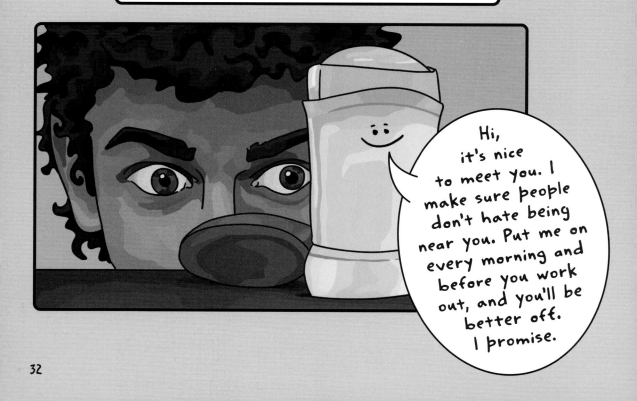

A lot of the other changes you undergo during puberty have some upside to them: muscles, manliness . . . . This "perk" really just makes your life a little more difficult. No one wants to suddenly start smelling bad. As long as you shower (*with soap!*) and use deodorant, this change is pretty manageable. It's probably a good idea to keep some deodorant in your backpack for gym days, sports days, or days when maybe you run to get to class on time. Make sure you get *deodorant*, which cuts or covers the smell, rather than *antiperspirant*, which inhibits sweating. Sweating is healthy and normal—you do want to sweat. You just don't want to stink.

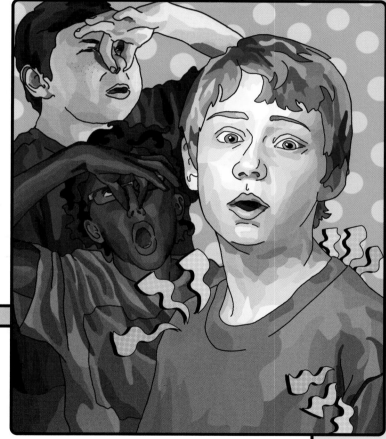

Speaking of stinking, be sure to wear socks. Your sneakers will start to smell *really* bad— so bad that you will kick off your shoes one day and wipe out everyone within whiffing distance. You will be wondering what rotting food or vermin could possibly smell that bad . . . and it will be your sneakers. Trust me—socks.

Who's the Guy with the BEARD?

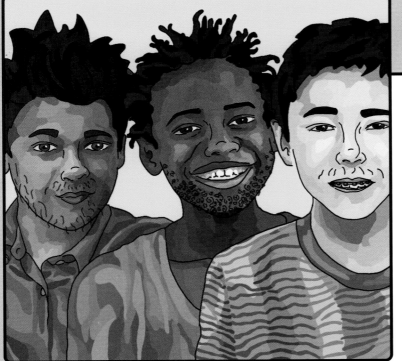

In addition to saying goodbye to your baby fat, and soft smooth skin, you'll also lose your round, sweet baby face during puberty. In what may feel like a fun-house mirror trick, your nose will get thicker, your chin will get longer, and your jawline will get more defined. The good news is, you will more closely resemble those comic book superheroes.

At the same time, prepare for the arrival of what may be the manliest touch of all. Facial hair is generally viewed as a pretty pivotal moment in this whole puberty experience. It's the most visible of your hair developments (unless you're going around showing people your crotch and armpits, which you definitely shouldn't be doing). Facial hair is probably one of the last changes you'll experience. And wow, does a sprinkling of hair across your upper lip make you feel manly.

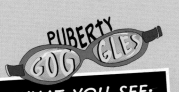

WHAT YOU SEE:

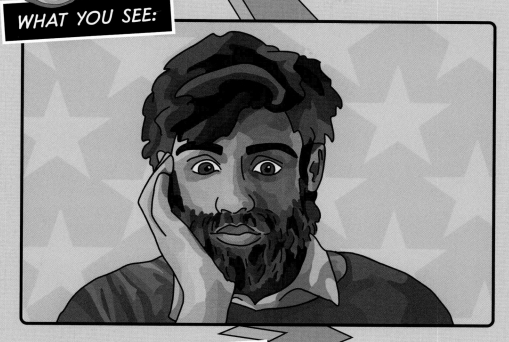

WHAT EVERYONE ELSE SEES:

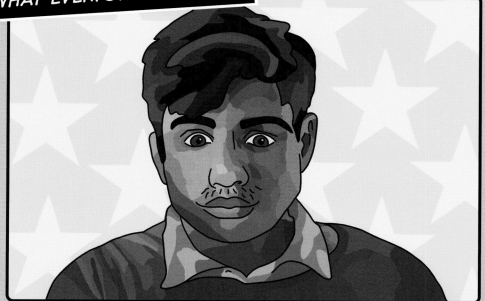

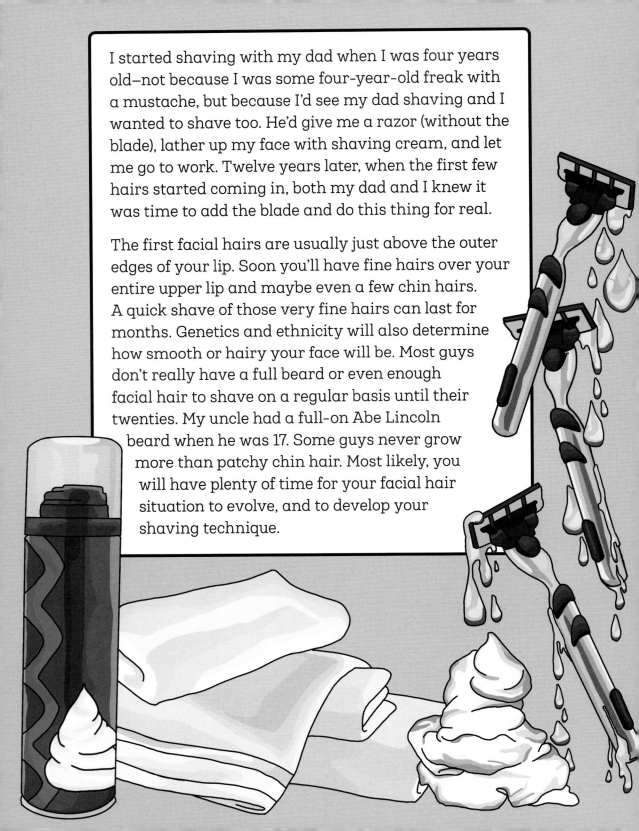

I started shaving with my dad when I was four years old—not because I was some four-year-old freak with a mustache, but because I'd see my dad shaving and I wanted to shave too. He'd give me a razor (without the blade), lather up my face with shaving cream, and let me go to work. Twelve years later, when the first few hairs started coming in, both my dad and I knew it was time to add the blade and do this thing for real.

The first facial hairs are usually just above the outer edges of your lip. Soon you'll have fine hairs over your entire upper lip and maybe even a few chin hairs. A quick shave of those very fine hairs can last for months. Genetics and ethnicity will also determine how smooth or hairy your face will be. Most guys don't really have a full beard or even enough facial hair to shave on a regular basis until their twenties. My uncle had a full-on Abe Lincoln beard when he was 17. Some guys never grow more than patchy chin hair. Most likely, you will have plenty of time for your facial hair situation to evolve, and to develop your shaving technique.

DIY SHAVING

Everyone has his own specific method for shaving, but here is the basic how-to:

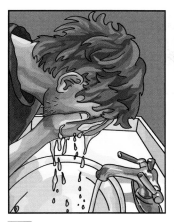

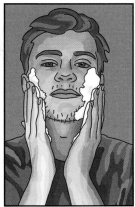

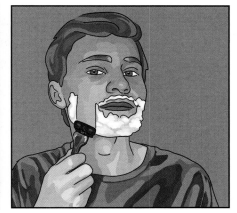

1. Wash your face with warm water. This helps kill off any bacteria that may be on your face, and the heat opens your pores, which makes it easier for the razor to catch the hair. A hot shower before you shave will also do the trick.

2. Spread shaving cream wherever there is hair on your face. Keep it out of your mouth and eyes, but be generous with globbing it around.

3. Using a new, sharp blade, start at the top and shave to the edge of your jawline with long and even strokes, moving further inwards with every stroke. The idea is to shave *with* the grain of your hair. Rinse the shaving cream and hairs off the blade after every stroke. It may take a few strokes to figure out the right amount of pressure so you are getting just the hair, not the skin.

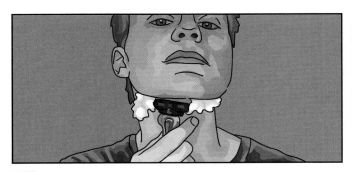

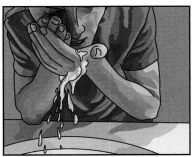

4. Shave below your jawline last, being really careful with your neck and under your chin. You may need to pull the skin tight and use shorter strokes in these tricky spots.

5. Wash your face with cold water to seal the pores.

Along Comes ACNE

Of all the indignities of puberty, acne may be the worst. It was for me. I let my acne affect my self-esteem, my confidence, and the choices I'd make. I would feel anxious if people looked too closely at me in school, I'd obsess over which creams and face washes to use. I let acne define me instead of being a temporary part of me. The bad news: About 80% of us experience acne during puberty. The good news: In most cases, it goes away once you get out of your teens.

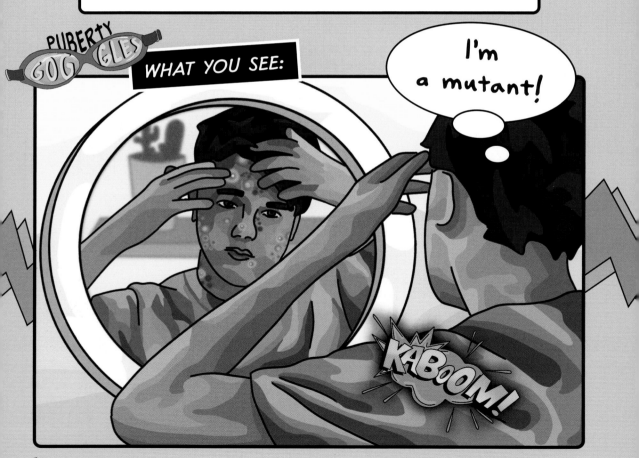

What causes acne? Like everything else that goes on during puberty, it's about hormones. The pores (hair follicles) in your skin contain *sebaceous glands*, or oil glands. These glands make *sebum*, the oil that lubricates your hair and skin so they look and feel good. Most of the time, your body makes just enough sebum to keep your skin healthy and working properly. But during puberty, the hormonal changes somehow overstimulate the oil glands, and you wind up all shiny and bumpy. Your pores get clogged with dead skin cells if there's too much sebum. Bacteria can get trapped inside too. All hell breaks loose in your skin—swelling, redness, whiteheads (clogged, closed pores), blackheads (open clogged pores), and pimples (clogged pores with bacteria in the mix). A zit with a puss-filled center? That's your body's reaction to the bacterial infection. It's all so nasty and unpleasant.

WHAT EVERYONE ELSE SEES:

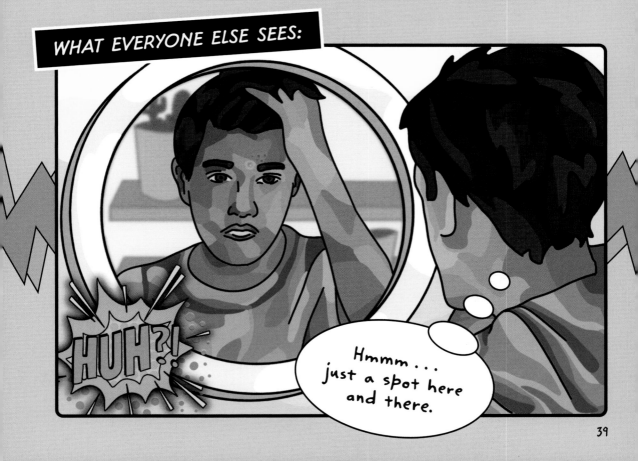

Zits

The best things you can do are also the easiest. Keep your face clean—wash with either a face wash or face soap and water twice a day. You don't want to use shower gel on your face. And don't touch the zits, as tempting as it may be. There are lots of facial cleansers and creams you can buy at the drugstore. Look for products with salicylic acid or benzoyl peroxide if you have breakouts or oily skin. One or the other will help, but they can also make your skin dry, so don't overdo it. If it gets really, really bad, you can also try a gel that contains adapalene.

If your zits look more like giant bumps or cysts, you should probably go to a dermatologist (a skin doctor). A doctor might prescribe a heavy-duty acne cream, or even an antibiotic to kill the bacteria causing the pimples. I went to a dermatologist at one point when it seemed like it would never end, and in my case, the antibiotic helped. I also changed some things in my diet—cut out soda, limited sugar—and used an array of natural products including tea tree oil. All of those things helped to varying degrees, but ultimately the thing that made the biggest difference was the passing of time. As puberty began to wind down and my hormones started to normalize, one by one, my pimples faded away. As awful as it can be, just remember that this, too shall pass.

KNOCK KNOCK. Who's There?

There may be some setbacks (cracks really) along the way, but, by the time you've made it through puberty, your voice will be much deeper. You'll go from sounding like a boy to sounding definitively like a man. You'll also have a newfound lump in your throat called the Adam's apple. This awkward protrusion must be really important right? Nope. It serves basically no purpose whatsoever. Guys get one and girls don't, so maybe that's something to brag about?

Testosterone causes a boy's larynx to get bigger and vocal chords to lengthen and thicken. This growth is what makes the Adam's apple pop out. It also causes the average boy's voice to deepen a full octave over the course of puberty. You don't just wake up one day with a deep voice the same way you don't just shoot up 6 inches overnight. It's a process, and your voice cracks while it goes through the deepening process. This can be embarrassing, but at some point, it happens to everyone so move on knowing that a dreamy, reliably deep voice awaits.

Who is Adam? And why is his apple popping out of my throat?

FREAK Show: PART 1

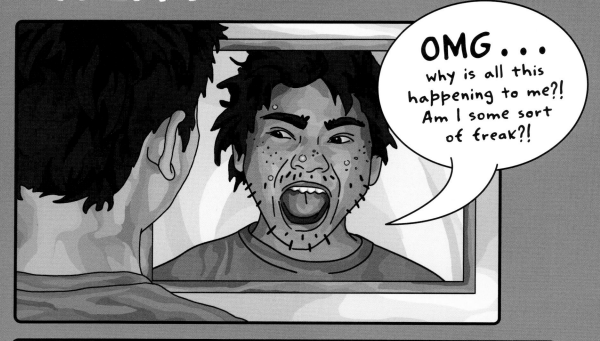

Calm down. You are not some sort of freak. At times, these changes can get overwhelming and cause people to panic. Why do some people start to worry about being a mutant during puberty though? It's probably because everything starts to look, sound, and smell different.

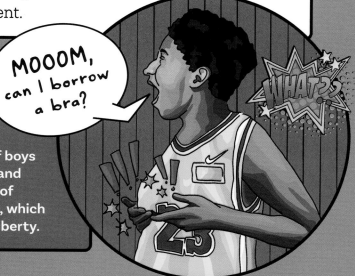

Are your **BREASTS** getting larger? Thought that was only supposed to happen to girls? It actually happens to as many as 70% of boys too. It's called gynecomastia, and it happens when your balance of hormones is thrown off a little, which happens quite easily during puberty.

Are you getting strange **LITTLE BUMPS** on your face (or elsewhere) that aren't zits? Welcome to the world of ingrown hairs! These can appear after shaving, or really any time, especially if you're on the hairier side. They're common, and easy to deal with: Wash with warm water, and then use sharp tweezers to pry the hair loose. Also be sure to use shaving cream when you shave.

Does your **HAIR** seem coarser, thicker, wavier, curlier, or kinkier? Hormones leave nothing untouched! My hair was always curly, but the curls tightened and my hair definitely got coarser and thicker when I went through puberty. Two of my brothers had straight hair that got really wavy. It's totally normal.

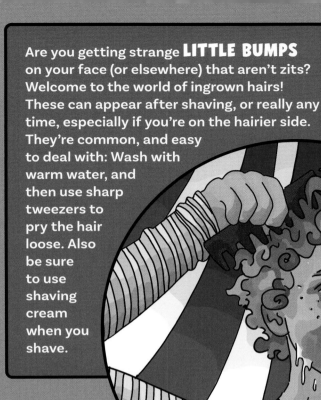

Mom and Dad—please don't send me to the circus.

Boys' **NOSES** have a growth spurt of their own during puberty. Like your arms and legs, your nose will grow faster than the rest of your body. While boys' and girls' noses are the same size until you're around 11 or 12, once puberty kicks in, boys' noses tend to grow bigger than girls. Puberty is also the time when little button noses might develop bumps that weren't there before. Think of it as developing character!

Good news: Whatever you're experiencing, you're probably not alone and whatever you're going through that's got you all worried, is perfectly normal.

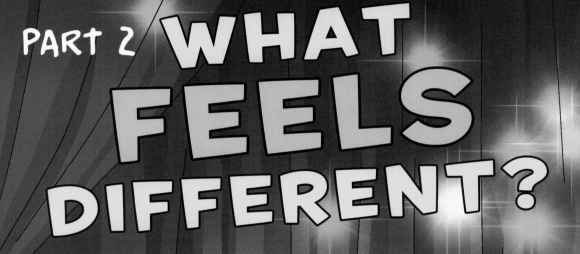

PART 2 WHAT FEELS DIFFERENT?

Your body (the outside) isn't the only thing that's changing. The same hormones that trigger physical changes, such as body hair and muscle growth, also drive emotional changes. Puberty gives you a nice grown-up body, right? Well, now it's time to mentally and emotionally grow into it.

As scary as pubic hair may be, just wait until you hear about love. You think acne makes you angry? Wait until your first pubescent fight with your parents. Your emotional development makes physical changes seem easy.

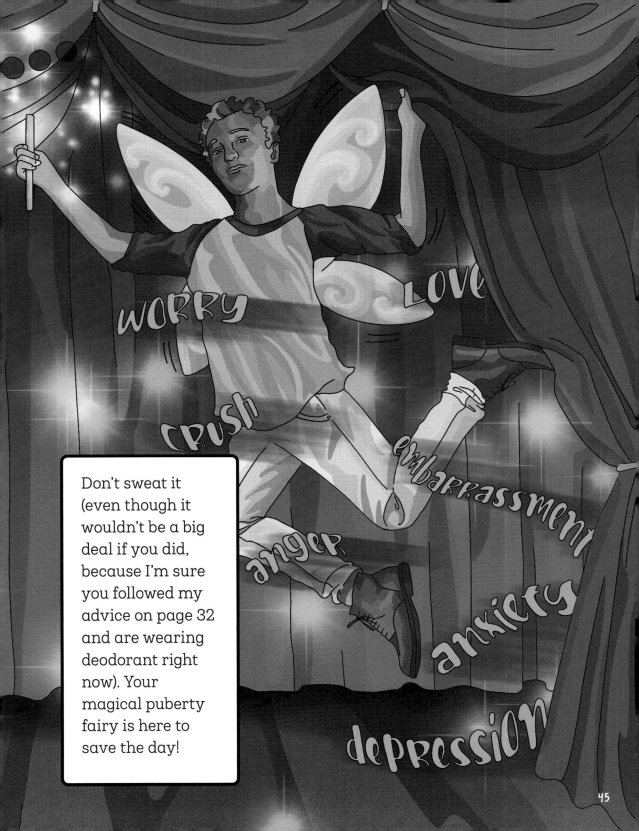

Don't sweat it (even though it wouldn't be a big deal if you did, because I'm sure you followed my advice on page 32 and are wearing deodorant right now). Your magical puberty fairy is here to save the day!

SEXUAL Feelings

One of the big, internal changes you'll notice is the development of sexual feelings. You go from "OMG, girls have cooties" to "OMG, girls have boobies" in a hurry. Remember how all those pages ago we talked about how your penis starts to produce sperm during puberty? Well, once your body starts producing sperm, you'll also start having sexual thoughts.

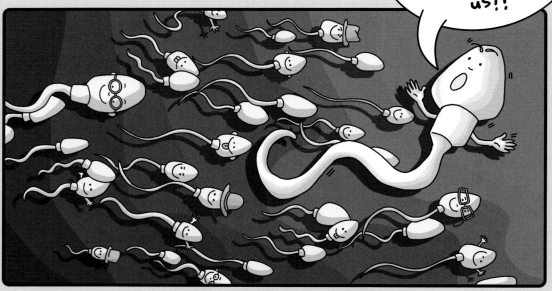

The development of these feelings means that you'll start feeling attracted to people and having sexual desires. It will all probably start with a crush on a girl or boy in your class or even a character on a TV show. (Katara from *Avatar: The Last Airbender* was my brother's first love.) And it only grows from there. My brother has crushes on real, non-cartoon people nowadays.

Starting to have sexual feelings and thoughts can feel weird and overwhelming. You might blush or feel self-conscious when you see your crush. You could get a stomachache, or think about that person (or people) all the time, even in your dreams. You may find yourself going out of your way in the hopes of running into that person. It can feel embarrassing if your crush is a friend or someone a lot older than you. I had a crush on a teacher once. My brother had a crush on his friend's older sister. You could find yourself attracted to a different person every single day.

You will inevitably do humiliating things around your crush. You could find yourself with a crush on someone who's not really thinking sexual thoughts yet. You could imagine that really hot camp counselor returns your affection, while she just thinks you're a cute little kid. You could even text your crush, like my brother did, to ask her who she likes—and have her father respond to you. All perfectly normal.

Sexuality:
THE CONTINUUM

Along with the development of sexual feelings, come feelings of sexual preferences. This is the time when you start to figure out whether you prefer girls, boys, both, or neither. And just to be clear, boys can like girls, boys can like other boys, and boys can like girls and boys. Some boys prefer one gender but are open to both. Some boys don't have any sexual feelings at all during their teens. Some people are really clear about their preferences early on. Others may go back and forth over the course of their entire lives. There is no right or wrong answer when it comes to who you love, are attracted to, and want to spend time with.

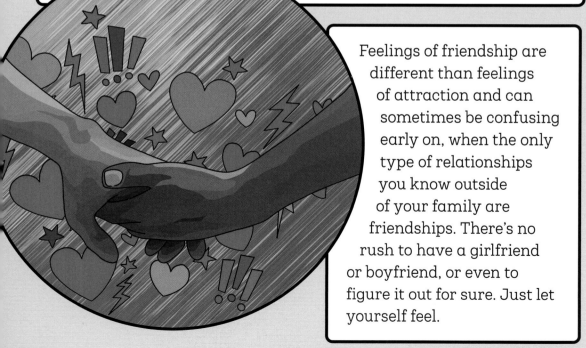

Feelings of friendship are different than feelings of attraction and can sometimes be confusing early on, when the only type of relationships you know outside of your family are friendships. There's no rush to have a girlfriend or boyfriend, or even to figure it out for sure. Just let yourself feel.

Though the majority of boys you know are probably attracted to girls, lots of boys (probably around 10%) are attracted to boys. It is normal and common to have same-sex feelings. But it can be challenging if you live in a place or are part of a family that doesn't understand that. And it can be stressful for people to have to hide their feelings. I have gay friends who grew up in New York City and felt completely comfortable about their sexuality as early as middle school. And I have friends who grew up in more conservative areas and didn't come out until college. It's really important that whatever sexual feelings you have, you don't feel ashamed.

HIS, HERS, AND THEIRS

The sexual organs you are assigned at birth determine your gender at birth. If you are born with a penis, you are considered a boy, and if you're born with a vagina, you're considered a girl. But not everyody feels at home in their body or identifies with the gender they are assigned at birth. Some people don't identify as a boy or girl, but something in between, something non-binary. People who don't identify with their gender assigned at birth are called trans. If you are trans, you probably have a different set of concerns as you go through puberty. If you are feeling any confusion about your gender, or anxiety about going through puberty, you should discuss this with a parent and/or your doctor or therapist. I am not an expert in gender identity, but if you are questioning yours, I can tell you you're not alone.

Erections Here, Erections There, Erections EVERYWHERE!

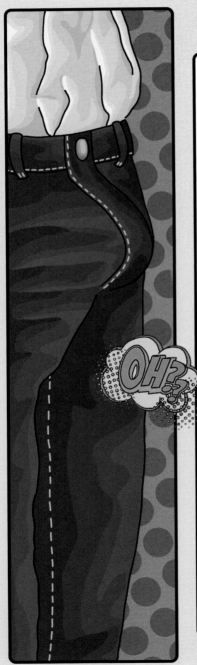

At the peak of my pubescent days, with my hormones revved up and raging, I certainly felt strange and self-conscious. One of the reasons for my embarrassment was that I didn't understand why my penis kept getting hard. Was it slowly evolving into a bone? Was it some sort of defense mechanism?

Turns out, my dirty little brain (just kidding, my totally normal, healthy brain) was thinking sexual thoughts. But not all the time. Sometimes during puberty you can get erections just because. You could be doing your ELA homework or playing basketball or walking to school, and not thinking sexual thoughts at all.

Whatever is going through your mind when this happens, your penis becomes hard because blood starts rushing to it. And as it fills with blood, it becomes harder. This probably sounds very formal and scientific right now, but trust me, when it's happening to you, it can be more than a little distressing.

I'll never forget little sixth grade me, helpless to the hormones raging throughout my gangly body, riding on the bus thinking about Princess Leia, or sitting in math class and getting excited by the curviness of certain circular numbers. Sound familiar? Suddenly you have to squirm in your seat, cross your legs, or put your backpack on your lap to hide your unwelcome and uninvited boner.

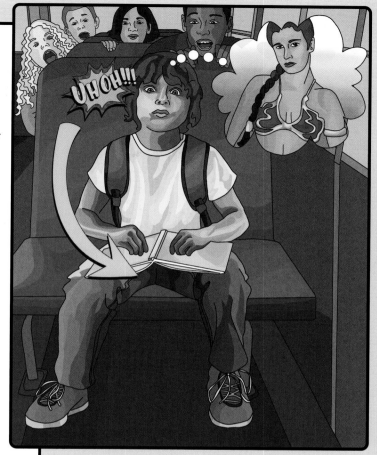

Erections will be a part of your life for a long, long time. But rest assured they are at their most relentlessly, surprisingly present while you're in the midst of puberty.

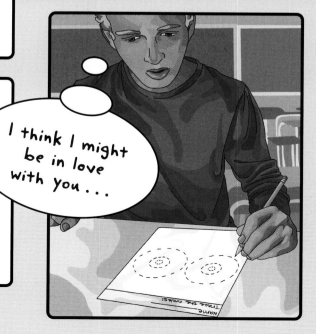

The Magic of MASTURBATION

One of the new routines you will likely develop once you start to have sexual feelings is masturbation. What's masturbation? I don't know, just go to Google Images and see what you can figure out . . .

JUST KIDDING! DON'T DO THAT!

I remember being in fifth grade, and some weird old dude in his fifties came into our health class to talk about masturbation. I don't know how one gets the job of being a masturbation guest speaker for children, but this guy had the lousy job—and he was bad at it. He was infuriatingly vague, telling me and the other boys in my class that "there was a part of your body you could touch that could cause you to orgasm." We spent all of snack time that day trying out different body parts. Maybe if I tug my ear upwards, maybe if I poke my belly button (after all I'd never really understood its purpose), maybe, maybe I could find the magical orgasm button.

A "HANDY" MASTURBATION GLOSSARY

ORGASM
When you reach a sexual climax and ejaculate.

EJACULATION
When semen comes out of your penis.

SEMEN
The sticky liquid that comes out of your penis when you orgasm (and ejaculate). Semen carries your sperm in it.

I don't want you to have to waste any of your valuable snack times pinching random body parts trying to unravel the mystery of masturbation. So here's the deal:

Masturbation is when you simulate sex with your hand on your penis. Like anything else, people develop their own specific preferences and variations, and that's for you to come up with and for me to never have to think about. This isn't shaving. The last thing I need is a bunch of middle schoolers following my step-by-step directions on how to masturbate.

Also, just so you guys know (and in case you've heard one of these other terms used), masturbating is called many wonderfully creative things such as jerking off, wanking off, wanking, jerkin' it, and rubbin' one out.

I know people who masturbated as often as possible in fifth grade, and I know people who didn't masturbate until they were in college. The fifth grade master of his domain and the college jerker-offer are both good, cool, normal guys! There are no rules when it comes to masturbation, and it's not something you want to force. If this isn't something you've heard about or that's been on your mind, great, file it away for a little while. Just know that there is no shame in masturbating—it is a totally healthy and normal part of your sexual development.

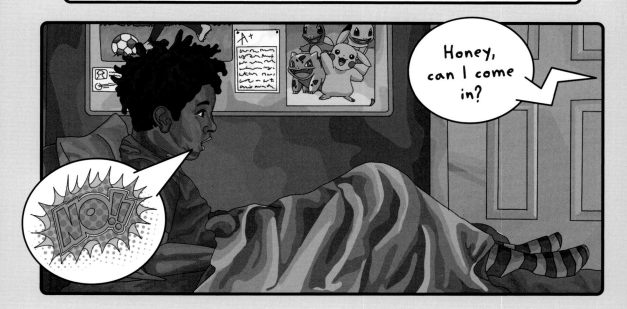

WET Dreams

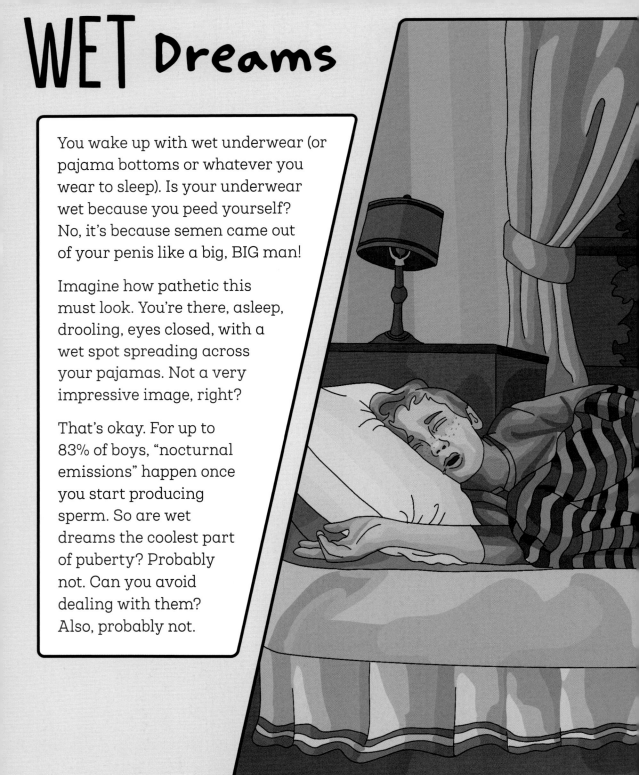

You wake up with wet underwear (or pajama bottoms or whatever you wear to sleep). Is your underwear wet because you peed yourself? No, it's because semen came out of your penis like a big, BIG man!

Imagine how pathetic this must look. You're there, asleep, drooling, eyes closed, with a wet spot spreading across your pajamas. Not a very impressive image, right?

That's okay. For up to 83% of boys, "nocturnal emissions" happen once you start producing sperm. So are wet dreams the coolest part of puberty? Probably not. Can you avoid dealing with them? Also, probably not.

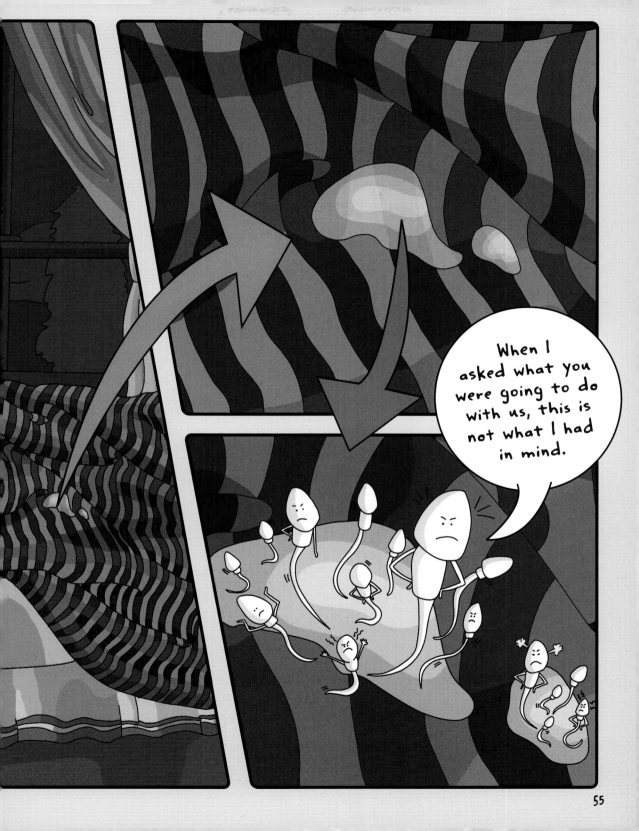

MOOD Swings

Puberty isn't all erections and wet dreams—it has its ups and downs. And mood swings—when you feel very happy about something one minute, and then, a moment later, you feel really upset by the very same thing—capture the highs and the lows better than any other aspect of puberty. Once again, our old friend testosterone is to blame. All the testosterone pulsing through your system can cause uncontrollable mood swings.

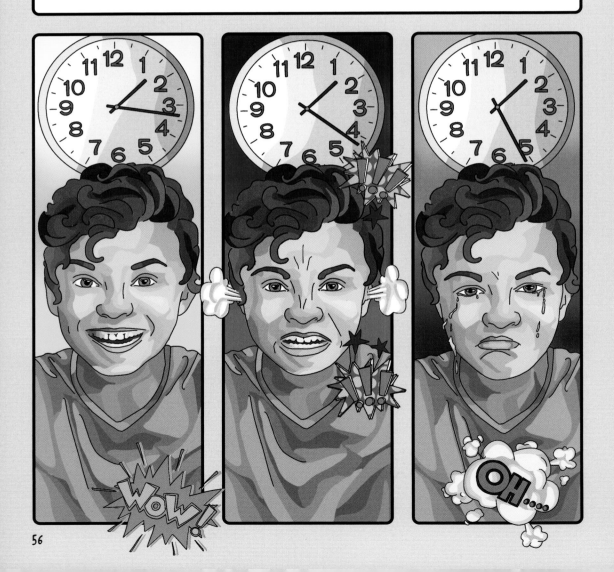

Mood swings can be confusing and disorienting not just for you, but for the people you interact with—your parents, siblings, and friends. Mood swings can be really upsetting. You may feel like something is wrong with you. (Nothing is wrong with you.) There's so much that's changing and happening that feels like it's out of your control. Honestly, the worst part about puberty is the degree that so much of your life is changing and you're not really getting that much of a say. You don't get to decide when your mood will turn dark any more than you get to decide when you're going to have your growth spurt or when your armpit hair will appear.

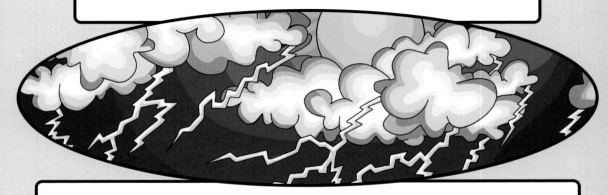

My advice on this could be applied to puberty as a whole. You can't control what's going to happen, but you can control how you react to your experiences. Accepting things as they are and taking it easy on yourself no matter what will make your life a lot less stressful. This doesn't mean that it's fine to go yell at people and freak out for no reason. It just means that this is a hard time, and not everything is going to work out the way you want it to. Your skin will most likely break out. Your crush may not return your feelings. And you might get inconvenient erections.

DON'T DRIVE YOURSELF CRAZY OVER THINGS YOU CAN'T CONTROL.

ANGRY Humans

One of the moods you'll find yourself swinging towards more and more often, is anger. You know that cliché about the angry brooding teen? It's a cliché because it's true. All that testosterone really brings out your anger.

You wouldn't know it now, but back in the day (all those five or six years ago), I had quite the temper. When my mom once told me I couldn't go to a concert until I finished my English paper, I threw a Wiffle ball bat across the living room. When my dad said I couldn't watch TV, I hid the remote from the whole family. If my mom asked me how my homework was going? Forget about it!

One time, I opened my mom's laptop to do my homework (we shared a laptop then), and I saw she had been googling "teenage anger." That really set me off. How dare she try to figure out what the hell was wrong with me!

Am I proud of that behavior? No, I am not. Have I learned from that behavior? Yes, for sure. I thought I'd make a chart to make your life easier.

DON'T	DO
• throw things	• try deep breathing
• yell at people	• go for a walk
• punch holes in walls	• exercise
• refuse to talk to people	• talk about your feelings

There are some strategies you can use to actually help prevent angry outbursts, and avoid walking around feeling angry all the time. Think about the things that make your blood boil, and try to avoid those triggers. And when you do get angry, pay attention to things that help you get over it. It might be listening to music or going for a bike ride. Meditation and mindfulness can really help too! (It's not just for monks!) There are three simple things you can do at the beginning of each day, before you go to sleep, or whenever you're feeling like you are going to explode.

Breathe deeply, in through your nose and out through your mouth, for several minutes.

Imagine a happy place (just not too happy or you might get a boner), or even try to clear your mind while you're quiet and breathing.

Make a list of three things (other than masturbating) that make you happy. You can write this list down every day.

These mindfulness basics can provide a sense of calm in the midst of all the constant chaos of puberty.

PARENTS: The Enemy

As you were probably able to tell from the fact that my mom not only googled "teenage anger" but downloaded a "How to Deal with an Angry Teenager" PDF, my parents and I didn't always get along while I was going through puberty. We disagreed about how often I had to go to school, how late I could stay out on the weekend, how clean my room needed to be, and so much more. Having now had a few years to reflect and also watch my parents deal with my brothers during their crazy years, I have some thoughts on the matter.

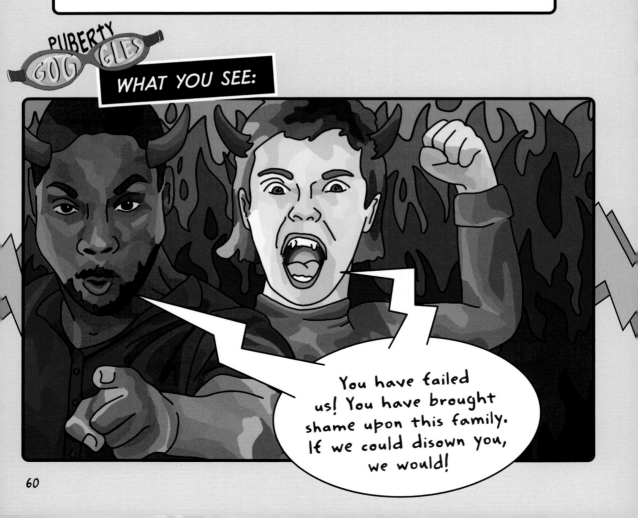

Are you and your parents going to fight sometimes? Yes. Is that okay? Yes. Their job isn't to be your friend, it's to raise you. During puberty, you want full control over your life. The teen years are all about breaking free from your parents and asserting your independence. That's basically your job. It's also your parents' job to keep you safe, provide boundaries, and make sure you're set up for future success. So regardless of what you may think and how much you may believe that you "hate" them or don't need them and just wish they'd leave you alone, know that it's probably not as bad as you think it is and your puberty is a difficult time for all of you.

WHAT'S ACTUALLY HAPPENING:

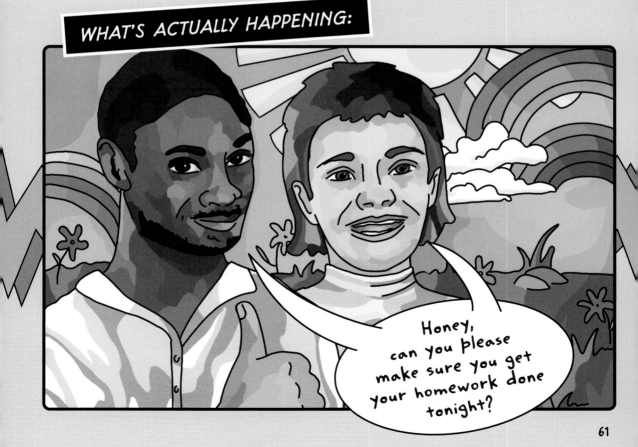

THRILL Seeking

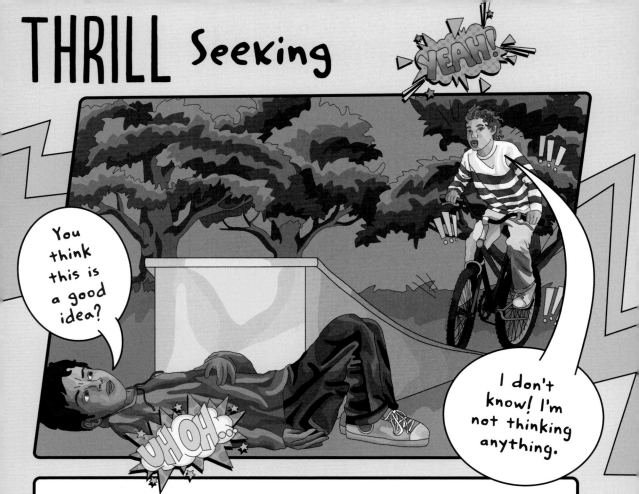

One of the many reasons we still need people looking out for us when we're teenagers is because teens are inclined to do risky and dangerous things. They think it's cool and fun. Well, let me tell you, there's nothing cool or fun about dying.

I've always been incredibly cautious so this wasn't a huge issue for me. I wish the same thing could be said about my brothers. All of them, while going through puberty, seemed to have some kind of a death wish. Whether it was riding a bike around New York City without a helmet, standing too close to the edge of the subway platform, throwing sharp projectiles at each other (at close range), climbing towering trees, or strolling to the center of a frozen pond to see if it was *really* frozen, they've all been reckless.

Lots of teens are reckless, and boys tend to be more reckless than girls. It's because the frontal cortex of our brains is not fully developed, and without it, we have trouble understanding the consequences of our actions. So we do what we want to do in the moment, not worrying about the next moment, or the next. Some of us behave this way well into our twenties. Not naming names.

Sounds dangerous? Well, it is. So I need you to fight every instinct your not-yet-fully-developed-brain has, and actually think before you act. Just take a minute to imagine what might happen if you decide to skip your algebra test or ride your scooter really fast around a blind turn. And do the smart thing—the thing that leaves you with a bright future instead.

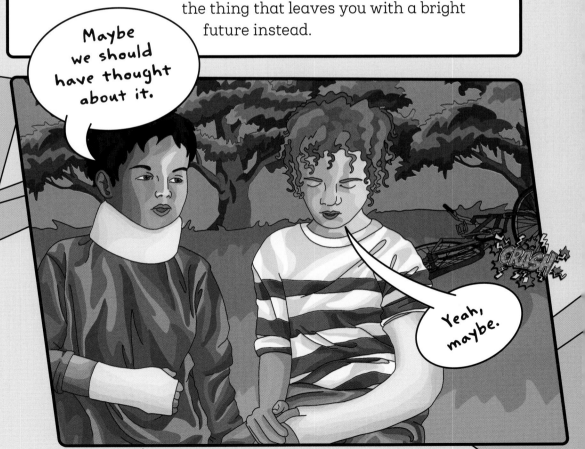

Why Don't I Like the Things
I USED TO?

Change is a defining part of puberty. One aspect of the full-body renovation is that you may not have all the same interests that you did before. Sometimes, people even change friend groups during this time.

In elementary school, I loved playing basketball. It was one of my main hobbies. I had a killer jump shot (I was like Stephen Curry before Stephen Curry was Stephen Curry). Once I got to middle school though, I lost my desire to play. I still loved watching basketball but didn't feel as strongly about playing it.

My best friend from elementary school and I stopped hanging out for four years! (Don't worry, we've become close again). My brother stopped playing Dungeons & Dragons and started to spend all of his time making amazing art.

FSSST

Another brother stopped playing the drums and took up Thai boxing. I know people who weren't social at all before puberty who then grew huge circles of friends. I know people who struggled in school and then started excelling and vice versa. These shifts can take many forms.

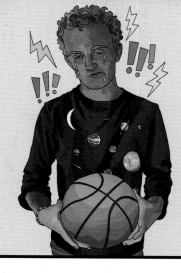

When something that's been one of your main pasttimes stops being a part of your life, it can be scary and weird.

But trust me, even though for so long basketball was my go-to activity and then suddenly I didn't really want to play anymore, it all worked out. I felt lost for a little while, but then I developed a new habit.

I started writing. And to this day, it's one of the big passions in my life. I also started playing basketball again, though not as often as I used to. Experimenting with new people and pastimes is part of figuring out who you are, or what kind of man you're going to be.

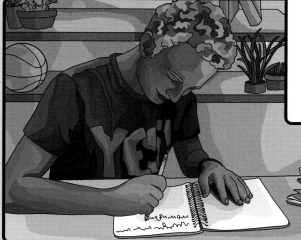

STRESS and ANXIETY

With new development, comes new responsibilities. Having real responsibilities for the first time (no offense to the betta fish you fed every now and then when you were in preschool) can be stress-inducing. School, social life, and family dynamics can be a lot to deal with over the course of these transformative years.

Dealing with more schoolwork, time management, social pressure, and chores—or even a job—can be stressful. Stress is when you feel overwhelmed or like you have too much to handle.

hobbies
SCHOOL
Love
SLEEP
HAIR
Popularity
Work
PARENTS
FRIENDS
Height

Organization is one area in which girls are generally far superior to us. There are exceptions, but in general, we walk around like moronic slobs while they keep everything neatly organized. "To Do" lists are actually really helpful. So are schedules: keeping track of what you need to do each day and each week can help you to manage your tasks and responsibilities and will definitely help reduce stress.

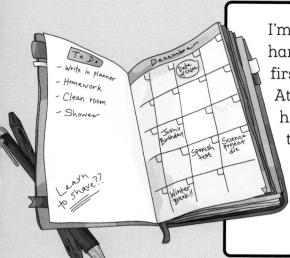

I'm not judging you if you don't use these handy tools, though. I think I made my first to-do list and schedule last year. At the beginning of middle school and high school the teachers would hand out these color-coded planners, and I don't think I used mine even once. In turn, I was stressed out about schoolwork all the time. Don't be like me. Plan, organize, and make your life easier!

Anxiety is related to stress but has some subtle, important differences. Anxiety is a feeling of worry, nervousness, or unease that you're experiencing about an event or person. It may feel like a stomachache or a racing heart, or just a sense of doom. I get anxious a *lot* and it does not feel good. But it's also incredibly common.

Different things can make people anxious. Large groups make some people tense, while others find one-on-one hangouts stressful. Some people have test or academic anxiety. For others, it's more social.

When it comes to managing anxiety, different strategies work for different people. Some people like deep breathing or visualization (imagining yourself in a peaceful, happy place). Others find talking about their anxiety with a therapist to be helpful. If you suffer from anxiety, then part of your puberty process will involve figuring out the best ways to manage it. Just know that most of the people your age are feeling anxious as well, often about the same things that worry you.

DEPRESSION

Like anxiety and stress, depression is really common during puberty. Depression is the persistent feeling of sadness and often results in a loss of interest in things that used to make you happy.

Rates of teenage depression, suicide, and anxiety are at all-time highs. In the next section, we will talk about the outside world and how things like bullying and social media impact your life. Depression is often a side effect of comparing yourself to others on social media, or a result of being bullied or excluded. Depression can be triggered by many things when you're a teenager. Here, now, we're just going to talk about how this makes you feel.

Depression can feel overwhelming and disorienting while you're in the throes of it. It can feel like it will go on forever, like things will never get better, or like you're all alone, feeling horrible. This isn't true though. You will come out the other end and you'll feel like yourself again. It may be in a few hours, or a few days, or even a few weeks. But your sadness will lift.

I'm not going to sit here and tell you that everything will always be light, breezy, and easy. It won't be. You're not a little kid anymore. Your new freedom and maturity and feelings bring with them new struggles and sadness. But these struggles can be overcome.

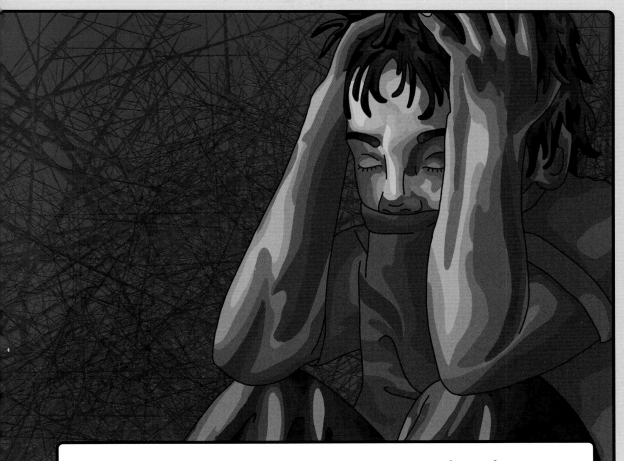

Depression can be triggered by your overactive puberty hormones. Sometimes, depression is the result of a chemical imbalance in your brain. Certain people are constructed in a way where their brain chemistry leaves them feeling sad. For people like this, there are medications to lift them up and balance their moods. If you think this may be your problem, you will need to see a psychiatrist.

Sometimes, depression is related to a difficult life event, like the death of a loved one, or divorce in the family. Sometimes, it's the result of a lot of anxiety and stress that becomes too much to handle. No matter what causes your depression, there are ways to get help—and it's really important that you do.

COPING WITH STRESS

If you're feeling overwhelmed by life in general, or schoolwork in particular, try changing your mindset. Instead of thinking "Holy crap, I'll never get all of this homework done," try thinking, "I'm going to start by doing one assignment, and then I'll try another assignment."

SLEEP! Getting a full night's sleep and having a regular sleep schedule can mprove your brain functioning and your mood, so make sure you're getting plenty of sleep!

DON'T BEAT YOURSELF UP. Telling yourself that you're such a loser for failing that test, or losing that point for your team will bring you down even more. Instead, remind yourself that it's just one test, and you'll study for the next one. It's just one play, and you'll have lots of chances to score.

CONGRATULATE YOURSELF FOR DOING A DECENT JOB. Don't demand perfection. In real life, nobody is expected to do everything perfectly.

FIND HEALTHY WAYS TO RELAX. Pet a dog. Listen to music. Take it easy when you're feeling tense.

WHAT TO DO WHEN YOU'RE DEPRESSED

- If you're comfortable, talk to a parent about it.
- Talk to a school counselor. They are trained to help.
- Talk to a therapist. (A parent or school counselor can help you find one.)
- Try to communicate with a close friend about what you're going through.
- Write, draw, or find another creative outlet that allows you to express your feelings.
- Be kind to yourself.

There have been many times in my life, particularly during middle school and high school, when I felt depressed. Those times have mostly passed, but the struggle goes on. Seeing a therapist or a counselor is a great way to stay on top of your mental health if you can find someone you like, and if your family can afford it. To this day, I still see a therapist every week. Sometimes, I'm just talking about how my week was and what's been on my mind, and other times, if I'm in a funk or feeling down we talk about what I can do to turn that around. There's no shame in struggling or in asking for help. This stuff is hard and no one should have to feel like it's on them to handle it all alone.

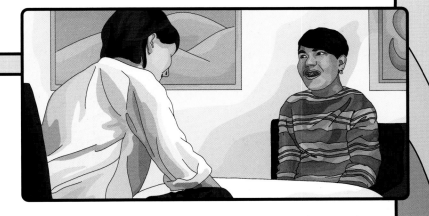

If you are having frequent nightmares, or want to sleep all day, don't want to go to school or leave your house, and have lost interest in the things you used to enjoy, you should definitely talk to a school counselor or therapist.

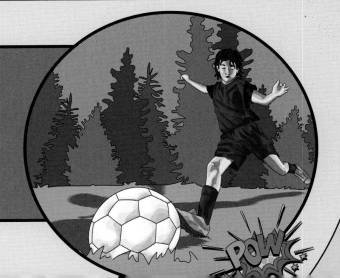

- **Exercise.** When you exercise, your body releases hormones, called "endorphins," which make you feel happier.

FREAK Show: PART 2

Everybody experiences different sexual feelings and moods. Pretty much anything goes during this crazy time of your life.

Am I a FREAK if...

. . . I MASTURBATE TOO MUCH? Probably not. Take it from me, you can masturbate A LOT without it being too much. It really only becomes "too much" when it starts interfering with your life—like if you cancel plans with friends, are being caused physical pain by it, or skip homework to devote your time to masturbating.

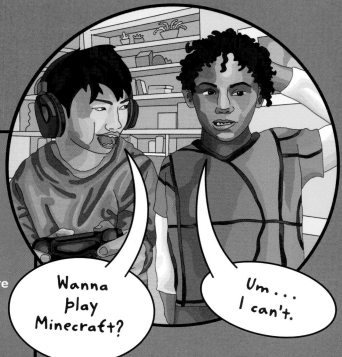

. . . I LIKE BOYS AND GIRLS? No. No. No. A million times no. There's nothing wrong with that whatsoever.

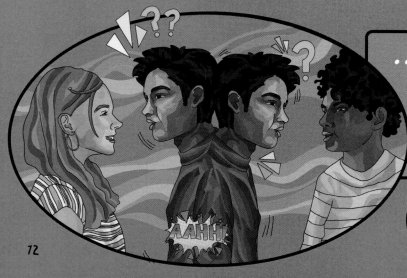

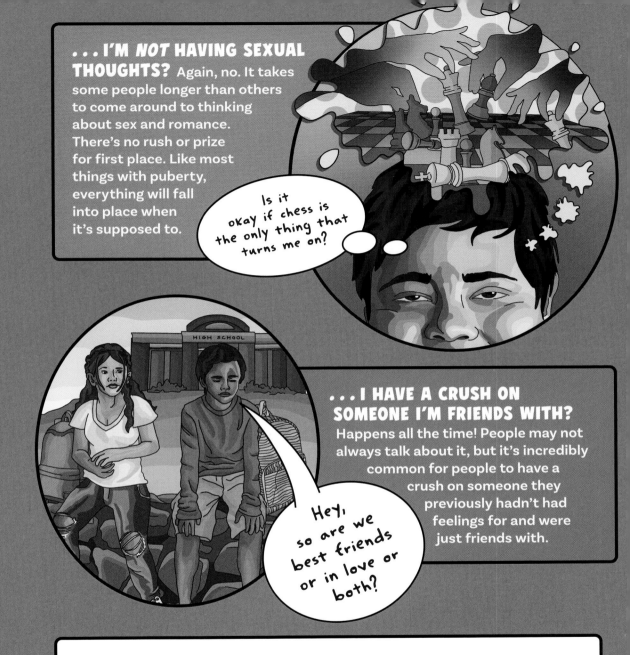

. . . I'M *NOT* HAVING SEXUAL THOUGHTS? Again, no. It takes some people longer than others to come around to thinking about sex and romance. There's no rush or prize for first place. Like most things with puberty, everything will fall into place when it's supposed to.

Is it okay if chess is the only thing that turns me on?

. . . I HAVE A CRUSH ON SOMEONE I'M FRIENDS WITH? Happens all the time! People may not always talk about it, but it's incredibly common for people to have a crush on someone they previously hadn't had feelings for and were just friends with.

Hey, so are we best friends or in love or both?

Welp, there you go! A little glimpse into all the ways you'll start to feel different as you start to look different. I know it can sound overwhelming and like there are a lot of downsides to puberty, but those are really just growing pains. When you come out the other side, you'll be a remarkable and impressive adult, inside and out!

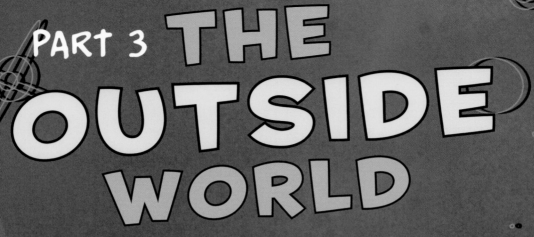

PART 3 THE OUTSIDE WORLD

A NEW WORLD

Welcome to our final segment of the book, Part 3, the grand finale. In the first parts of the book, we discussed how you'll look different and how you'll feel different as you go through puberty. We've talked about YOU. Now, it's time to talk about everyone else (which may be hard, I know).

How do you think about other people?

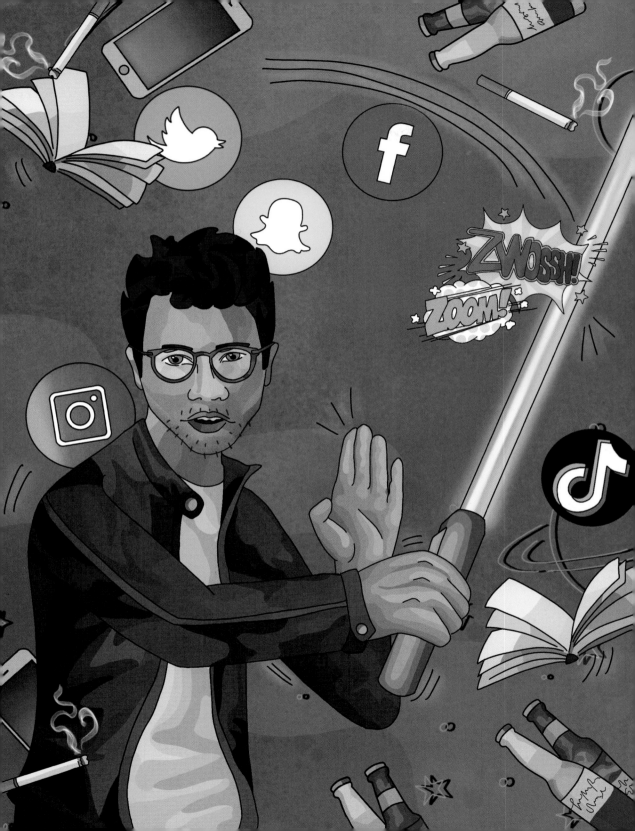

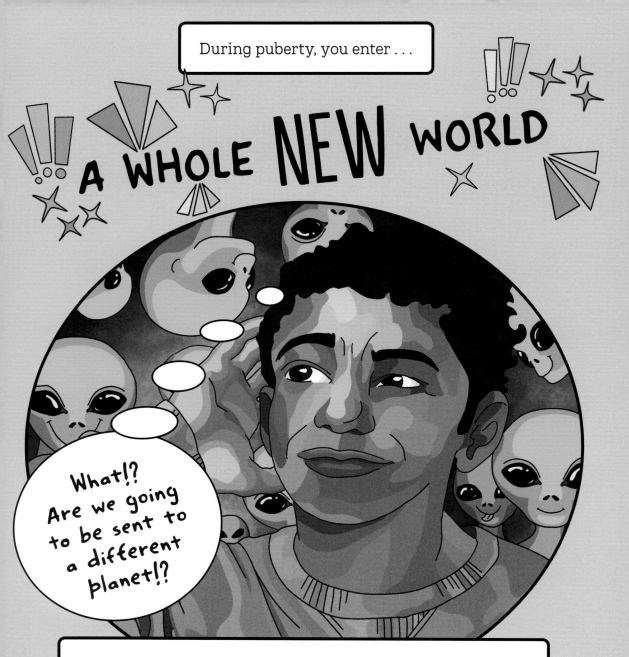

During puberty, you enter . . .

A WHOLE NEW WORLD

What!? Are we going to be sent to a different planet!?

No. Not like that. This world is just a different place for adults than it is for kids. In this section, we'll talk about the specific challenges the outside world will pose while you go through puberty—as well as some of the challengs you'll face in your new, grown-up life.

Whether you realize it or not, for much of your pre-pubescent life you've been protected. Your family has kept you safe. You've been sheltered because, for most of your childhood, you probably haven't had your own phone or computer, or easy access to a tablet or other device. You haven't had very much unsupervised time. You've lived in the world that the adults in your life have curated for you, picking out what they thought was safe and suitable. Unfortunately, we're not all Peter Pan, so we can't stay young forever. You probably didn't always notice and appreciate all the outside control. Maybe you thought, "I'm not a baby! I can do whatever I want!" more than once—or every single day.

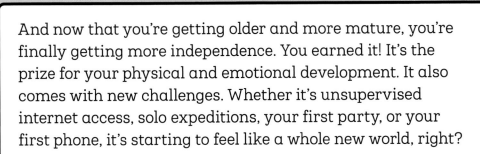

And now that you're getting older and more mature, you're finally getting more independence. You earned it! It's the prize for your physical and emotional development. It also comes with new challenges. Whether it's unsupervised internet access, solo expeditions, your first party, or your first phone, it's starting to feel like a whole new world, right?

What's the best way to navigate it? Just be true to yourself. The problem? That's not always as easy as it sounds.

Under (PEER) Pressure

First, if you don't already know it, look up the song "Under Pressure" by Queen (it's amazing), and you'll appreciate my little header above so we can move on with the book.

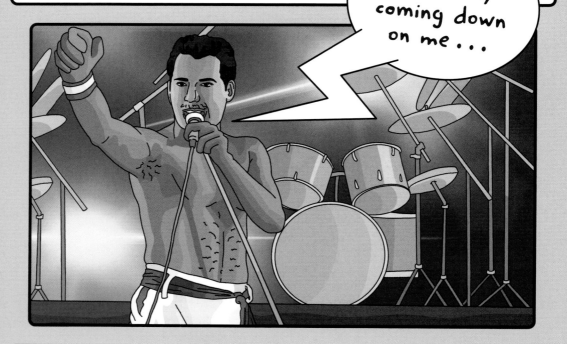

Under pressure, coming down on me . . .

One of the biggest reasons why it's not always easy to "just be yourself" is peer pressure. Most of the bad decisions you'll make while going through puberty you'll make because of peer pressure. Sometimes peer pressure is very straightforward. Friends or classmates will urge you to do something you're not so sure about. Other times, it won't be that obvious. Peer pressure also comes into play when you do something because you *think* your peers expect it from you and you don't want to disappoint them—you want to fit in.

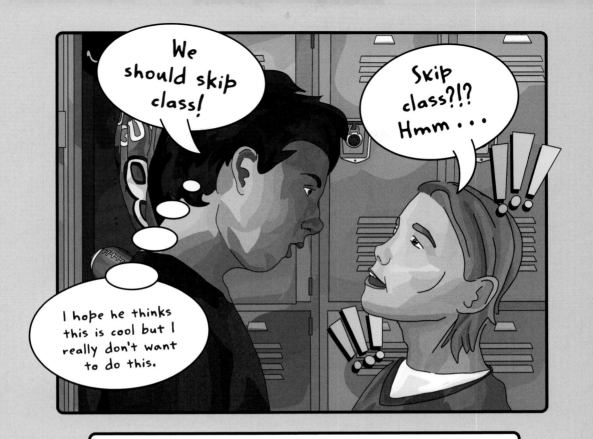

When it comes to peer pressure, you're facing an uphill battle. My grandmother used to ask me, "If you were standing on the top of the Empire State Building and one of your friends told you to jump, would you?" To this, I'd say "How close of a friend?" I'd only say this to annoy my grandmother. In actuality, I understood her point. Don't do something stupid, something you don't want to do, just because someone's telling you to do it.

I get that it's not always easy to avoid "jumping" when your friend says "jump," so I have a few pieces of wisdom to share with you:

CRUSHING Peer Pressure

1. More often than not, your friends are probably just as scared or hesitant as you are. They just think that YOU will think cutting class or sipping on a beer is cool, so they do it even though they may not want to. The solution to this problem is easy. Communicate. If you're honest and open about what you're not comfortable doing, your peers are more likely to be honest and open about the things they're not comfortable doing too, and that will help all of you make sure you're not pressuring one another.

2. If you, as a teenager, with your barely developed frontal cortex and zero sense of repercussions, actually think something is a bad idea, you probably shouldn't do it.

3. Try to be a good influence on the group. Don't be the guy who other kids' parents don't want to have over. Better yourself and your peers by speaking up and leading by your wise example.

4. Make sure you're not pressuring. Sometimes, you can be pressuring someone without realizing it. Peer pressure doesn't always come from a bad place, and it's not always obvious. Sometimes it's as simple as you wanting your friend to enjoy something you're doing, or you not wanting to do something alone. In high school, one of my friends kept trying to get another friend to try a puff of a cigarette. The smoker wasn't doing this to be mean, he just wanted company and thought our friend might like it. He was wrong. Years later, the non-smoking friend told us he'd found it really upsetting. Sometimes, even when your intentions aren't bad, you can still be making someone uncomfortable. So just make sure you're not pressuring anyone into doing something they don't want to do.

Be cautious, be aware, be true to yourself, and remember: Friends who don't accept you for who you are, aren't truly your friends. Surround yourself with people who encourage you to do the things you want, not ones who force you to do things you don't want to do.

RISKY Business

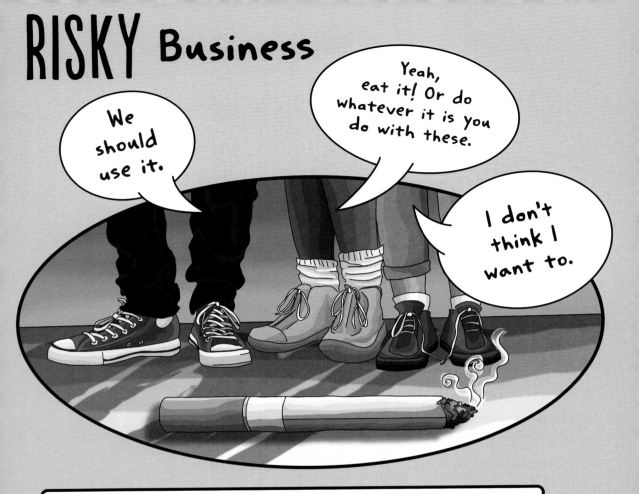

The teenage years are when many people first experiment with alcohol and drugs. Peer pressure certainly plays a role in this. You will almostly definitely feel pressure to try drugs, drinking, smoking, or vaping because so many other people are doing it or trying it out.

Here's the thing. I've been there. I'm not going to sit here and tell you to "just say no" or anything like that. This is not a rule book. However, it is full of my recommendations. So, staying true to that, I'll make some recommendations.

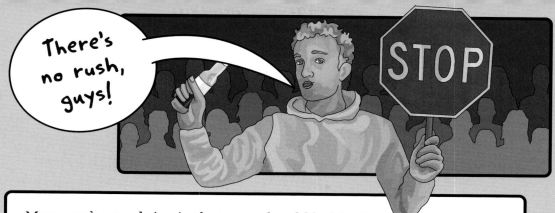

My very best advice is that you should hold off as long as you can. Some people will want to try drugs and drinking in high school. Others may start to partake in college. Some people don't do anything until after they've hit the legal drinking age. And some people never try drugs.

One of my coolest uncles didn't have a single drink until he was 24. One of my best friends tried smoking at 13. I love them both, and they're both awesome people. But, as my friend would now admit— he should have waited much longer. Your teenage self is making decisions that your adult body and brain have to live with.

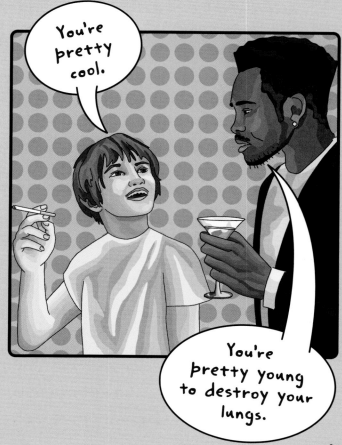

When you're in the midst of it all, it feels like there's pressure, like there's some rush to try drugs, to drink, to do it all. But there is no deadline. The vices will always be there. Once you're out of your teenage years, you will still have the rest of your life to legally drink or smoke if your fully developed brain decides that's something you want to do. Once your brain is more developed, you'll be better equipped to make decisions about these things. Plus, you will *never* regret waiting. But you will regret it if you try one of these things before you're ready and it backfires. So why rush it?

I am not going to tell you to never drink or do drugs. I am going to recommend that at a bare minimum, you wait. Why?

One time, at a party, one of my friends had a little too much to drink (okay, fine, it was way too much to drink). He left the party and was heading home on the subway and, the next thing he knew, he was at a subway stop an hour and a half away from where he lived. He had no idea how to get home. Because he'd had too much to drink, he'd fallen asleep on the train and missed his stop. He also woke up to a string of panicked texts and voicemails from his parents.

This became a story that we all liked to joke about and make fun of the friend for. The thing is, he put himself in a really dangerous situation. It ended up being okay, so it was a learning experience for that friend—and for the rest of us too. But there very easily could have been a different, more tragic ending to the story. There are real risks and downsides to experimenting with drinking and drugs at such a young age, and it's important to be mindful of that. You don't want to become one of the stories where everything doesn't turn out alright.

DRINKING, DRUGS, DOWNSIDES

Starting to smoke while you're still growing interferes with your growth. You want to grow big and tall, right?

Binge drinking between the ages of 12 and 17 increases the chance of mental illness and can lead to a decline in cognitive ability. You want to be smart, right?

Drinking and smoking weed (marijuana) or tobacco, can in some cases, lead to the use of more serious illegal drugs.

Your lungs are critical for success in athletics, and are really important for other things, like, you know, breathing.

Nothing good comes from teenagers drinking, smoking, or trying drugs. Plus, it's illegal. You can get into serious trouble.

SOCIAL Media

Your parents probably think social media is just some way to stay in touch with family and get into political arguments with distant friends. They may not understand what social media is for us.

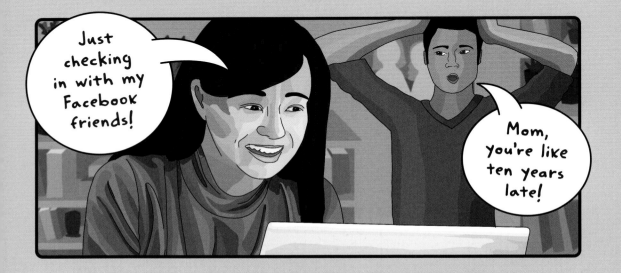

We've got TikTok and Instagram, Facebook and Snapchat, Twitter and a bunch of others. For our generation (yes, we are of the same generation), social media is a part of everyday life. In some ways, this is great. In other ways, not so much.

On one hand, social media has made it easy to connect with the world around you, to find people with similar interests, to discover new music, films and political beliefs. That's all great.

On the other hand, in study after study, social media has been definitively linked to an increase in depression and anxiety in younger people. Do I like seeing what my friends are up to? Yes. Do I like being anxious and depressed? No, not at all.

PUBERTY GOGGLES

WHAT YOU SEE:

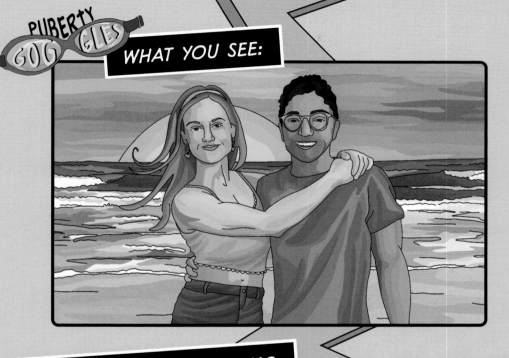

WHAT'S REALLY HAPPENING:

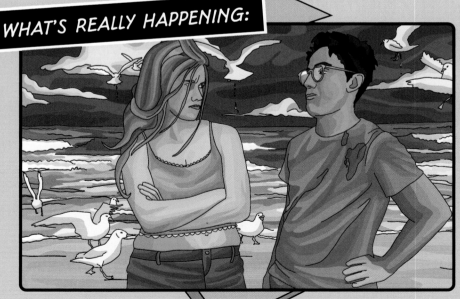

I get the appeal of social media. But there's also a tremendous downside. I've spent days feeling bad about myself because I saw how much fun it looked like other people were having when I knew I wasn't having nearly as much fun. I'll let you in on a little secret: No one's having as much fun as it looks like they're having. Social media is not real life. Real life is real life (this is that top-level insight I bring to the table) and interacting face-to-face, engaging with people in real life, that should be the priority.

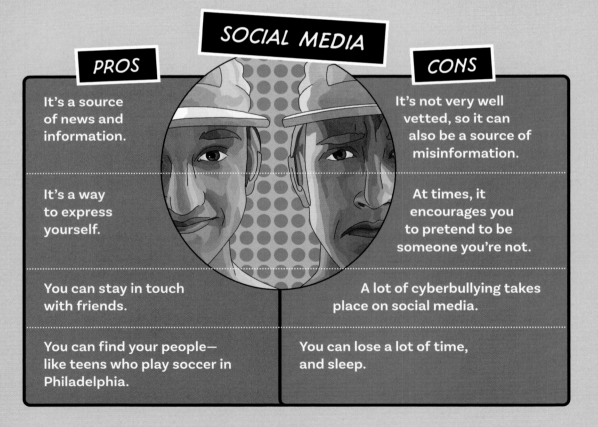

SOCIAL MEDIA

PROS

- It's a source of news and information.
- It's a way to express yourself.
- You can stay in touch with friends.
- You can find your people—like teens who play soccer in Philadelphia.

CONS

- It's not very well vetted, so it can also be a source of misinformation.
- At times, it encourages you to pretend to be someone you're not.
- A lot of cyberbullying takes place on social media.
- You can lose a lot of time, and sleep.

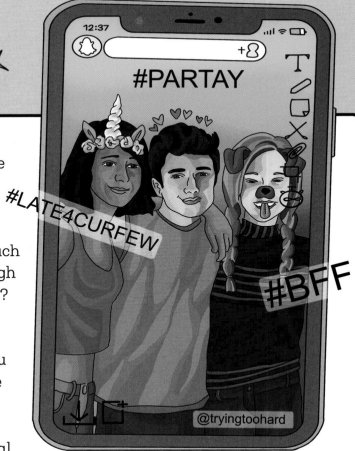

It's good to check in with yourself and see how social media is making you feel. Do you always have a knot in your stomach after scrolling through your Instagram feed? Do you feel anxious, like you're missing something, when you go on Snapchat? I've found it very helpful from time to time to step away from social media altogether. I call it a "social media cleanse," and I delete my social media apps for a week or two and let myself reset. It's also helpful to set limits on how much time you'll spend per day and per week on a screen and on social media. You can set the limits right in your phone. I'm not saying you have to forgo social media altogether. Just always make sure that you're maintaining a healthy relationship with it! A good rule for yourself is to make sure that you spend more time having conversations and doing things with real live people than you are spending on social media.

New Phone, WHO DIS?

Social media isn't the only way in which our upbringing is different than past generations. In the "olden days" (as my brother likes to refer to the eighties), people were not able to be in constant touch the way they are now. (Ask your parents about pay phones. Parents love to talk about pay phones.) Cell phones and texting were a complete game-changer. Now, we can't picture our lives without a cell phone, but it wasn't always that way. Texting is still a relatively new technology, and one that we should be sure we're making the best use of.

My parents had a simple mantra when it came to my phone and communication: "The only reason you have a phone is so you can communicate with us." I was given a phone when I started sixth grade, because that's when I started traveling to and from school on my own, and my parents wanted to be able to find me. I had to text them when I got to school to let them know I had made it. I had to let them know every time I left one place and arrived at my destination. Is communicating with your parents the coolest part about getting a phone? Absolutely not. But if you're good about communicating with your parents, they won't give you a hard time about anything else you do with your phone.

PHONE HOME

It seems easy (and it is). Yet, it is something I greatly struggled with. Once I started going out, I would hardly ever communicate with my parents about where I was and what I was doing. This would drive them crazy. I'd be out, having the time of my life, and my parents would be home, on the verge of a panic attack because they didn't know where I was or what I was doing.

Then, when I'd eventually come home, we'd fight and I'd end up grounded because I didn't text or call them to let them know where I was and what I was doing. This sequence of events would happen over and over again for years until finally, I discovered something life-changing. It cost me nothing to take the extra 30 seconds to text my parents, but that text meant everything to them. The best part about making this change was that we wouldn't fight, and I wouldn't be grounded anymore. I know it goes against every pubescent instinct you have, but your life will be a lot better if you PHONE HOME!

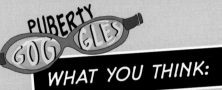

WHAT YOU THINK:

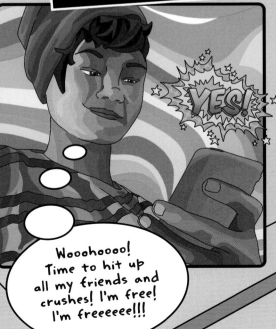

Wooohoooo! Time to hit up all my friends and crushes! I'm free! I'm freeeeee!!!

WHAT YOU REALIZE LATER:

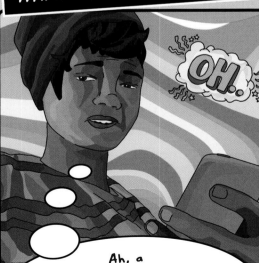

Ah, a device I have for the sole purpose of communicating with my parents and letting them know I'm alive and safe.

What is Cyberbullying?

Cyberbullying is when bullying or harassment takes place via technological devices (phones, computers, and any social media platform). Cyberbullying happens A LOT, and a big reason why is because it feels abstract. Because you're not actually saying these things directly to another person's face (you're just typing them), it's easier to not think about how you might be hurting or affecting the people you're talking to or about. Remember that even when you're communicating through texting or social media, you're still dealing with real people who have real feelings.

So . . . Nudes

Nudes are naked pictures people take of themselves or other people. Exchanging nudes can be common among high schoolers and, given how sensitive a topic this is, it doesn't get talked about enough. Also, nudes are most often shared digitally, which makes it even more important to handle them carefully, if at all.

THE BIG NOS OF NUDES

Ideally, you should not be exchanging nudes AT ALL. In many states, it is illegal to send or request nudes.

- Never pressure anyone to send a naked picture.

- Never send anyone a naked picture of yourself.

- Never, never, never, never share nudes that someone privately shares with you.

Internet PORN

This is one of those topics where you're lucky that you have me to talk to. The internet (or the "interweb," as your grandparents probably call it) has become the thing that everything else revolves around. We watch movies and YouTube videos on the internet. We find the answers to our most pressing questions, such as how many Kardashians there are, or whether everyone's pee smells weird after they eat asparagus. We look for information on famous people we're curious about, and we search for images from movies, sports, and events. It can be very entertaining.

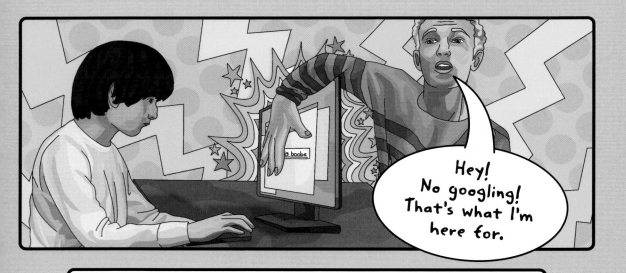

However, there are some darker parts of the internet as well. There is content that's inappropriate for people your age, and frankly, for people of any age. Always be careful about what you're looking up and how you're looking it up.

If you don't know what porn is, great! You can skip the next page.

Still here? Well, I'm not going to tell you not to watch porn. Similar to my approach to talking about drugs, I will *strongly* recommend holding off on it. A lot of bad things can come from watching porn. You may stumble onto images that you *really* don't want to see, and can't unsee once you do. But I'm also not going to tell you to never, ever do it, because I think that, at some point, you will probably check it out. You're not a freak for being curious.

So, if you're one of those people whose curiosity gets you googling (and you definitely don't have to be one of those people), here are some things to remember.

1. Porn is not what real life is like. (This is a good rule to remember about the internet in general.)

2. Most porn is bad, poor quality, and uninteresting.

3. The treatment of women can be really, really disrespectful and problematic at times.

4. If you wait until your twenties or thirties or whenever to experience porn, you will never, ever look back and think "I wish I'd started watching porn when I was 15." That will just not happen.

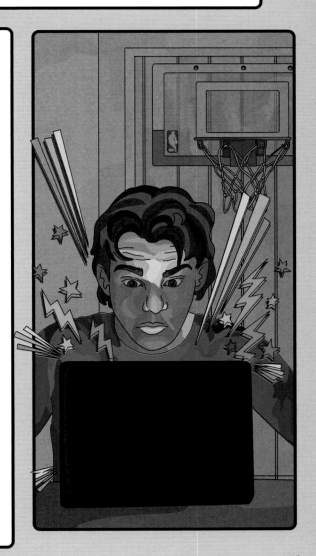

R-E-S-P-E-C-T

Not unrelated to the "porn talk" we just had, respecting women is a critical part of growing into a responsible man. There is a lot of sexism in the world, and a lot of it is really subtle. It's your job to confront and combat sexism, and not be a part of the problem. Just like it shouldn't be on people of color to fix racism, gender inequality should not be a woman's problem.

Sometimes, that means you have to make sure you're not taking up too much space and that you're leaving room for women, whether it's in the classroom or in casual conversations with your friends. Sometimes that means not spreading out your legs when you're sitting in a public space. And sometimes that means not taking part in demeaning conversations about girls' looks or personalities or intelligence or anything else. It means putting an end to those conversations altogether.

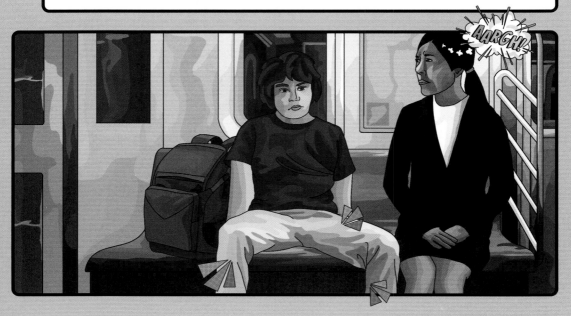

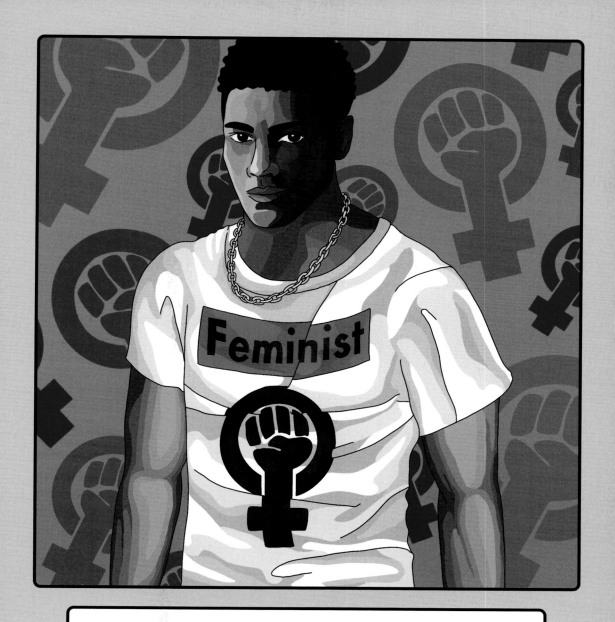

Being a feminist isn't some radical idea. It just means that you believe men and women are equal. It's really that simple. Be a feminist. Any time you see or hear or sense that girls and women are not being treated the way you would see boys and men judged or treated, do your best to speak up and actively shut down that behavior.

TOXIC Masculinity

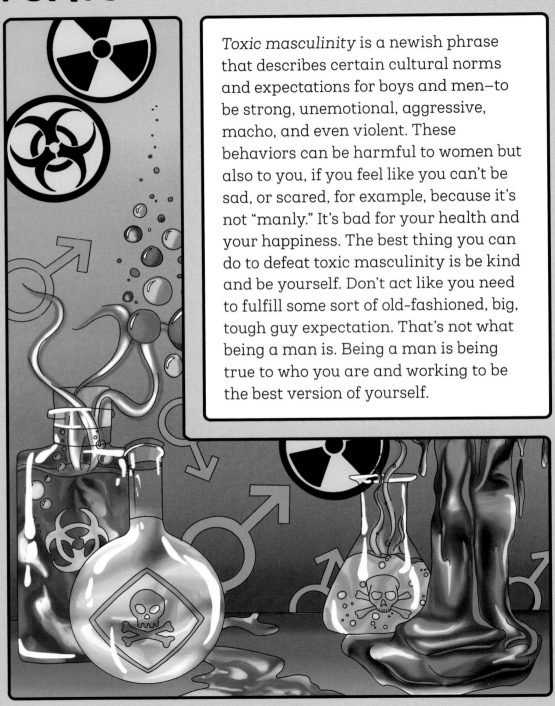

Toxic masculinity is a newish phrase that describes certain cultural norms and expectations for boys and men—to be strong, unemotional, aggressive, macho, and even violent. These behaviors can be harmful to women but also to you, if you feel like you can't be sad, or scared, for example, because it's not "manly." It's bad for your health and your happiness. The best thing you can do to defeat toxic masculinity is be kind and be yourself. Don't act like you need to fulfill some sort of old-fashioned, big, tough guy expectation. That's not what being a man is. Being a man is being true to who you are and working to be the best version of yourself.

MYTH: Men have to be athletic.

FACT: Men can be athletic, but they don't have to be. Men can be artists. Men can be teachers. Men can love politics and hate sports or love singing and despise wrestling. I love sports, but I also love art. I love singing (well, listening to other people sing at least) but am also always down for a quick wrestle with my brothers (don't tell my mom). Being a man doesn't mean you have to be put in a box. You get to embrace what you love, no matter what it is.

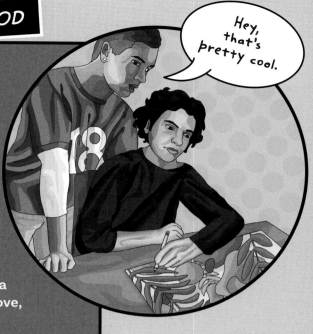

Hey, that's pretty cool.

MYTH: Men shouldn't talk about their feelings.

FACT: Men have feelings too, and there's nothing "manly" about not sharing them! It's healthy to talk to your friends and family about your feelings and about how you're doing. Keeping on a happy (or angry, or non-expressive) face can be exhausting, and can also lead to feelings of depression.

I'm feeling fragile today.

MYTH: It's cool to be mean.

FACT: It's cool to be nice. I don't know why, but there's this idea that it's somehow alright for guys to be mean. That it's the "cool" thing to do. It really isn't. Treat others the way you want to be treated. So many people complain about their teenage years and go on to say that the worst part is how "mean teenagers are." Hormones can make you temporarily meaner, and part of that meanness is about how other people act, but part of that is also up to you.

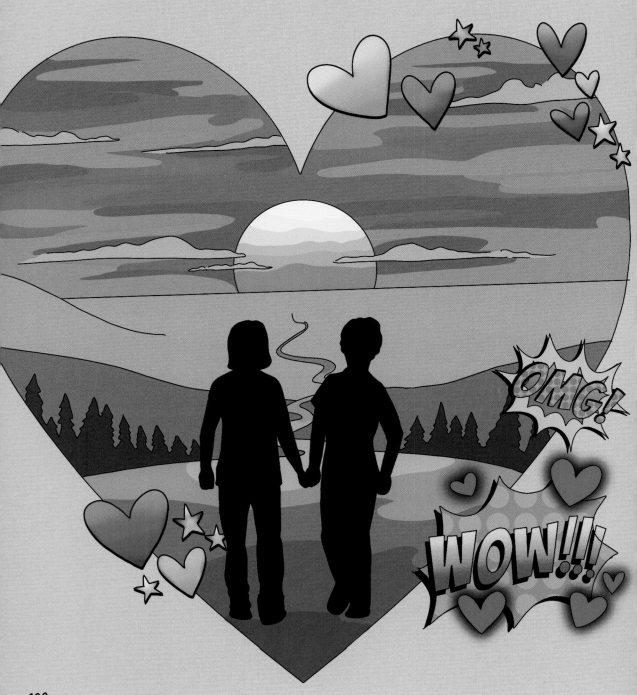

Not everyone has a romantic high school relationship, but some people do. If you are one of those people, it's really important to work to have a healthy relationship. Will it end in marriage? Probably not. But while it does last, it's worth making the effort to keep things positive.

What do I mean exactly by a "healthy relationship?" You have to respect each other, and a big part of that is respecting your partner's space and individuality. It's easy to get caught up in the fun of having a relationship and liking someone else and then lose sight of how you may be treating each other.

This is a time for you to be developing and learning about yourself and the world around you. Sometimes, when you're younger or new at it, a relationship can become all-consuming. Being in a relationship in high school can be a good opportunity to learn about yourself—if you have space for the individual growth you're both supposed to be going through during this time.

Set boundaries together in terms of what you're both comfortable with sexually. Get on the same page about how much time you want to spend together, either one-on-one or in a group. One of my friends had a girlfriend who *always* wanted to be with him—she would get mad at him if he had any other plans. She even wanted him to quit the baseball team! It was unhealthy, and he knew it, and he ended things with her.

School SUCKS

If you love school, God bless you. Working hard, participating in class, getting good grades, and joining extracurriculars will all serve you well in life. I did not love school, and I know a lot of people who felt the same way. Still, I'm going to be hypocritical and tell you that school should be a priority, because that's good advice.

What's really unfair about school at your age is that it actually matters. If it were up to me, middle school and high school would be a time for you to explore your interests and develop basic life skills with no stakes whatsoever.

Unfortunately, it's not up to me. So school does kind of matter. The choices you make will in one way or another influence your post-pubescent life. Your actions in high school will determine if or where you go to college, which in turn will determine the opportunities available to you when you are ready for "real life." Every time I skipped school or failed a class or did something stupid and unnecessary (and regretful), my dad would tell me that I was closing another window and cutting off my opportunities. I didn't see it then, but what I learned is that you can't avoid having to do a certain amount of schoolwork. You just postpone it. Take it from someone who spent the summer before college doing algebra in summer school, worrying that my college was going to rescind its acceptance. And don't do what I did.

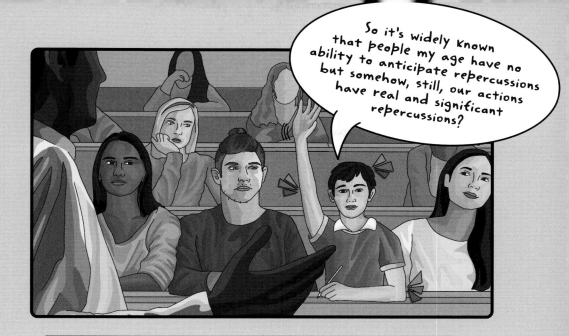

So it's widely known that people my age have no ability to anticipate repercussions but somehow, still, our actions have real and significant repercussions?

Since I graduated from high school, I've come up with some strategies that help me succeed in school. Being the generous and giving author that I am, I thought I'd share some of them with you:

SECRETS OF SCHOOL SUCCESS

MAKE SCHEDULES. Decide how you're going to spend your day before you sleep through most of it. It's totally fine to make time in your schedule for hanging out with your friends and relaxing, but also make sure you're setting aside time to do your work!

EAT LESS SUGAR! I could be locked in a Zen monastery and eating nothing but kale, and I would have a hard time focusing. However, eating less sugar does make a big difference. Cutting out candy and limiting my soda intake has really benefited my ability to focus.

LET PEOPLE HELP YOU. When I was younger and people would offer to help me, I'd turn them down, I thought "Hey, I'm a big boy, I don't need anyone's help!" That was so not smart. Since I've started letting people help me (teachers, tutors, even my parents!) and asking for help when I need it, I've done much, much better.

Alone @ LAST

Independence looks a little different depending on where you live. If you are growing up in a city (like I did) your newfound independence means that you're able to walk around by yourself, ride the subway or bus, and go to different neighborhoods. If you live in a suburb or more rural area maybe it means you can start learning to drive, and your friends (and you) may start having parties with little or no parental supervision. Wherever you are, you are entering a new era of independence, of you truly going off into the world by yourself.

As Uncle Ben said in *Spider-Man* (have I mentioned Uncle Ben?), "With great power, comes great responsibility." Being on your own is very cool and well earned! But, it means you have to be responsible, make good choices, stay in touch with your parents, and be careful.

If someone offers you candy to get into their van or car, say no. You should say no because candy is high in sugar, which isn't good for a developing child. Oh, and because they might kidnap you.

This may be a clichéd exaggeration, and many strangers are just good people who you haven't met yet, but there are also some bad eggs out there. And that's why it's important to listen to your parents! Once you get a taste of freedom, you may want to push your parents away, to think you're a big man who can take on the world all alone. Well . . . maybe hit the brakes a bit.

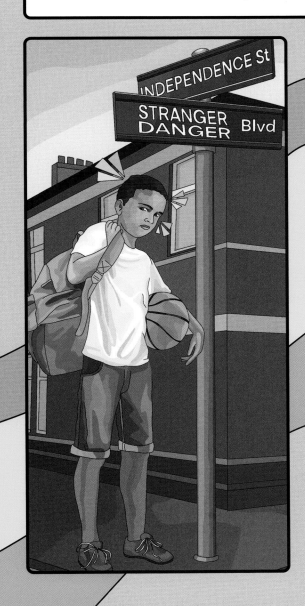

My brother used to play basketball with his friends every day after school. One day, he came home all excited that a man who had been watching them play told him that he should be a pro, that he was naturally gifted. The guy even offered to coach my brother. As someone who's spent a lot of time watching my brother play, I knew this was suspicious. My mother patiently listened to the story, told my brother he was an excellent basketball player, but that he should either find a different court, or not talk to that guy if he insisted on going back. (It turned out that our suspicions were right. Later that year, the man had to be removed by security because he kept inviting boys up to his apartment.)

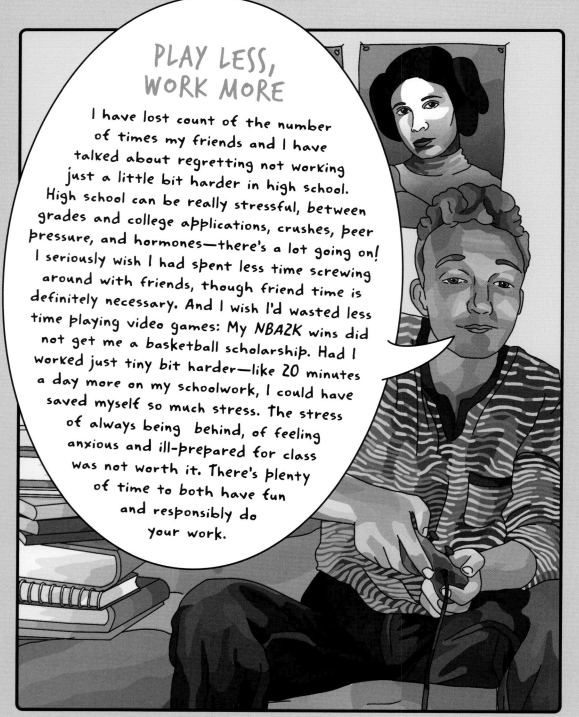

PLAY LESS, WORK MORE

I have lost count of the number of times my friends and I have talked about regretting not working just a little bit harder in high school. High school can be really stressful, between grades and college applications, crushes, peer pressure, and hormones—there's a lot going on! I seriously wish I had spent less time screwing around with friends, though friend time is definitely necessary. And I wish I'd wasted less time playing video games: My NBA2K wins did not get me a basketball scholarship. Had I worked just tiny bit harder—like 20 minutes a day more on my schoolwork, I could have saved myself so much stress. The stress of always being behind, of feeling anxious and ill-prepared for class was not worth it. There's plenty of time to both have fun and responsibly do your work.

BE HERE NOW

There's nothing I hate more than when I'm hanging out with my friends and everyone's on their phones. This may be the single worst norm of our generation. You're there, in person with a bunch of people, and you're all on your phones. WHY? Some Friday nights I'd look around while my friends and I were all gathered at a Chipotle or in someone's living room, and not a single person would be speaking or looking up from their phones. The thing is, especially when you're our age, it's easy to "unplug" for a little while. Now, when my friends and I hang out, we put our phones away. We check every hour or so but aren't glued to our screens. Instead, we're focused on hanging out and having fun. I really wish I started being better about unplugging sooner.

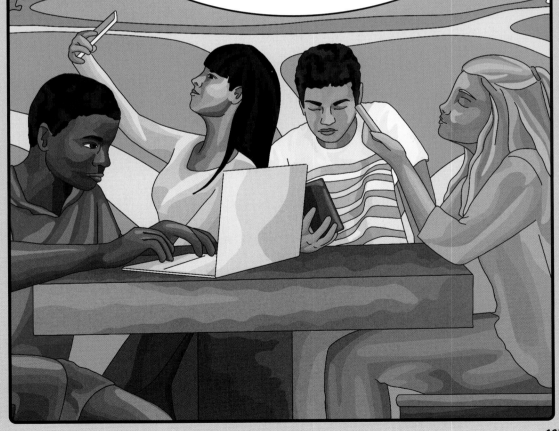

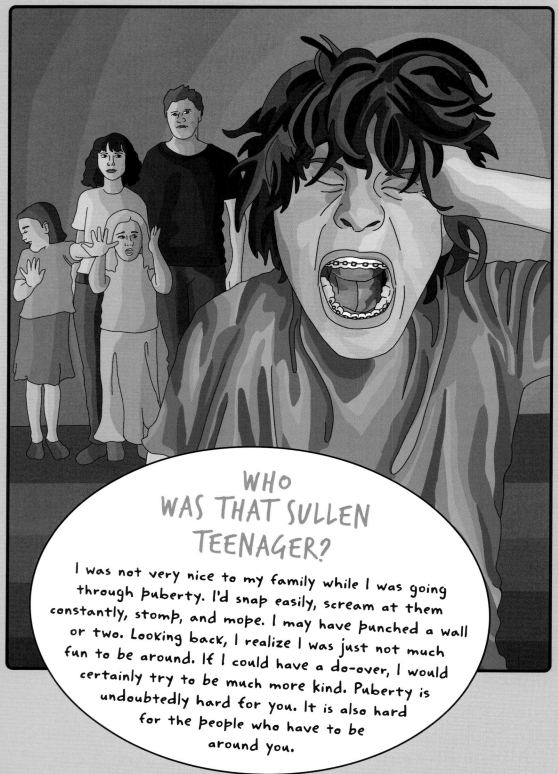

WHO WAS THAT SULLEN TEENAGER?

I was not very nice to my family while I was going through puberty. I'd snap easily, scream at them constantly, stomp, and mope. I may have punched a wall or two. Looking back, I realize I was just not much fun to be around. If I could have a do-over, I would certainly try to be much more kind. Puberty is undoubtedly hard for you. It is also hard for the people who have to be around you.

YOU & ME, We Are Family

As we come close to the end of our time together, I thought I should leave you with some words of wisdom. But unfortunately, I realized that I am in fact very unwise. So I decided to borrow some advice from my man-crush and absolute favorite person ever, President Obama. (When I have kids, I want to name one of them Barack.) In an address to graduating high schoolers, he spoke about the importance of community, and I want to pass along that lesson.

During these transformative years, you'll discover what you believe in, what matters to you, who you are, and what you stand for. This may not be as exciting as when your penis grows, but, it's much more meaningful. What does that have to do with building community? In President Obama's words, "No one does big things by themselves. . . . So be alive to one another's struggles. Stand up for one another's rights. Leave behind all the old ways of thinking that divide us—sexism, racial prejudice, status, greed—and set the world on a different path."

You've been gifted with a voice. How are you going to use that gift? You don't have to decide this minute. But have I mentioned Spider-Man's Uncle Ben?

FREAK Show: PART 3

At long last, our farewell is here. It's been one hell of a journey, and I'm sure you're as sad as I am to see it come to a close. Before we say goodbye, here's some final reassurance that you are not a freak.

Am I a FREAK if...

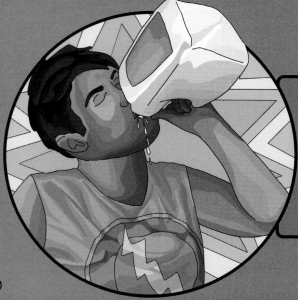

Me +Myself +i

...I DON'T DATE ANYONE IN HIGH SCHOOL.

No. In fact, I think I was a freak for dating someone at 16. Middle school and high school years are great for making friends and figuring out who and what you do and don't like. It's easier to accomplish those things on your own rather than when you're in a relationship.

...I DON'T DRINK OR TRY DRUGS.

No! Honestly, you're probably smarter than everyone else. You are not missing a thing and in the long run, your brain cells and your future self will thank you.

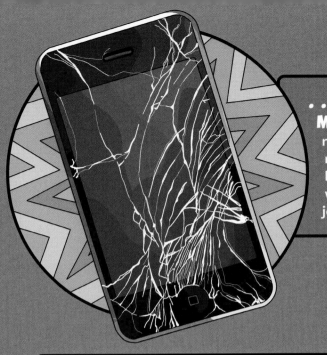

. . . SOCIAL MEDIA MAKES ME FEEL LONELY. This could not be less freakish. Social media makes *everyone* feel lonely. Try real connections with live people. They get the job done.

There you have it! It's a wrap! Are you a man yet?

Remember, no matter how scary and weird puberty may seem while you're going through it, it does come to an end, you're not alone, and you're definitely not a freak!

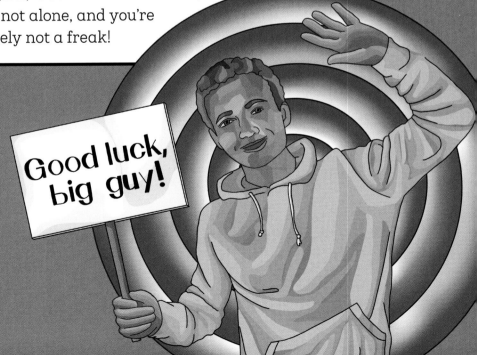

Good luck, big guy!

RESOURCES

Since you may not have a big brother, and definitely should not be googling, check out these resources if you want more information on a specific subject.

GENERAL PUBERTY INFO

amaze.org

healthychildren.org

Insight Into the Teenage Brain, TEDx Talk by Adriana Galván

kidshealth.org/en/kids/boys-puberty.html

plannedparenthood.org/learn/teens/puberty

Questions Every Teenager Needs to be Asked, TEDx Talk by Laurence Lewars

teenhelp.com

youngmenshealthsite.org

MENTAL HEALTH

Confessions of a Depressed Comic, TEDx Talk by Kevin Breel

MentalMusic podcast

My Anxious Mind: A Teen's Guide to Managing Anxiety and Panic by Michael A. Tompkins and Katherine Martinez

teenlineonline.org

thetrevorproject.org

SUBSTANCE ABUSE

newportacademy.com/resources

projectknow.com/teen/resources

SAMHSA.gov

teens.drugabuse.gov/teens